Advances in Mesopotamian Medicine from Hammurabi to Hippocrates

Cuneiform Monographs

VOLUME 37

Advances in Mesopotamian Medicine from Hammurabi to Hippocrates

Proceedings of the International Conference
"Oeil malade et mauvais oeil,"
Collège de France, Paris, 23rd June 2006

edited by
Annie Attia and Gilles Buisson

with the collaboration of
Markham J. Geller

BRILL

LEIDEN • BOSTON
2009

This book is printed on acid-free paper.

Library of Congress Cataloging-in-Publication Data

International Conference "Oeil malade et mauvais oeil" (2006 : Collège de France)
Advances in Mesopotamian medicine from Hammurabi to Hippocrates : proceedings of the International Conference "Oeil Malade et Mauvais Oeil", Collège de France, Paris, 23rd June 2006 / [edited by] Annie Attia and Gilles Buisson.
p. ; cm. – (Cuneiform monographs, ISSN 0929-0052 ; 37)
Includes bibliographical references and index.
One chapter in French.
ISBN 978-90-04-17876-2 (hard cover : alk. paper)
1. Medicine, Assyro-Babylonian–Congresses. I. Attia, Annie. II. Buisson, Gilles. III. Title. IV. Series: Cuneiform monographs, 37. 0929-0052 ; [DNLM: 1. History of Medicine–Ancient Lands–Congresses. 2. History, Ancient–Ancient Lands–Congresses. WZ 51 I605a 2009]

R135.3.I58 2006
610.9–dc22

2009022060

ISSN 0929-0052
ISBN 978 90 40 17876 2

PRINTED IN THE NETHERLANDS

CONTENTS

AVANT-PROPOS

Jean-Marie Durand

L'étude de la médecine ancienne a toujours été une des sources de sa recherche pour un de mes glorieux prédécesseurs au Collège de France, le professeur René LABAT, car il en avait, non seulement la compétence, mais le goût. Les textes médicaux représentent de fait un corpus qu'un spécialiste de notre discipline peut difficilement éviter, s'il veut avoir une connaissance complète du Proche-Orient, au moins celui du Ier millénaire, eu égard à son importance numérique et, surtout, aux possibilités qu'il offre de mieux entrer dans la connaissance de l'idéologie et de la science mésopotamiennes. Ces « vieilles gens », préoccupés par des maladies ressenties avant tout comme signes de la colère de leurs dieux, y trouvaient matière à une inquiétude qui allait bien au delà du souci immédiat de « rester en bonne santé ». Dès l'époque ancienne, au moment des textes de Mari, c'était déjà vers le devin, le *bârûm*, que l'on se tournait pour lui demander la cause d'une maladie, lequel répondait laconiquement y voir la marque de l'intervention d'une divinité, conseillant d'aller se présenter à elle. Le « médecin », l'*asûm*, était alors surtout un praticien qui « rafistolait » la partie malade, et il avait plutôt les apparences de notre ancien « chirurgien ». Cependant, dès cette époque c'était dans le jardin du même devin que l'on pouvait trouver telle plante médicinale rare, ce qui montre chez cet individu l'union du souci religieux et de la recherche scientifique, ou au moins le souci d'une médication efficace.

Lorsqu'au Ier millénaire, on constate désormais dans les bibliothèques publiques ou celles des techniciens l'existence de vastes pharmacopées et de maints rituels religieux avec leurs incantations et leurs manipulations de produits, il faut tenir ce résultat pour attendu. Dans leur souci de réparer l'offense aux dieux les Mésopotamiens avaient manifestement fini au cours du temps par s'organiser et aboutir dans la recherche des plantes et autres produits naturels, ainsi que dans celle de leurs combinaisons, qui leur permettraient de s'arranger avec cette mauvaise humeur divine et d'en pallier les effets.

Ces impressionnantes pharmacopées et ces recettes de toutes sortes qui les combinent sont, faut-il l'avouer, une joie pour le philologue, grand amateur de mots, et nos dictionnaires ont enregistré dans leurs colonnes maints produits de cette recherche. Cependant, par de là la satisfaction de recenser les noms des maladies, se fait aussi sentir le besoin de les identifier à celles d'aujourd'hui; par de là le patient recensement des médications, se manifeste la préoccupation d'en connaître l'efficacité, ce qui devrait conduire sinon à les reproduire, au moins à en identifier les éléments. Ces beaux soucis se heurtent au fait que, tant pour les plantes que pour les pierres, les descriptions que nous en ont laissé les Mésopotamiens sont surtout impressionnistes et relèvent plus de la « chose vue » que d'un examen minutieux ou d'une classification botanique précise. Sans compter que, de nos jours, bien des espèces ont dû disparaître ou se modifier. L'obstacle majeur vient aussi du fait que, souvent, l'« amateur de mots » ne sait pas toujours de quoi ils parlent et se trouve créer des nomenclatures qui font sourire praticiens et spécialistes de la machine humaine ou animale.

Je n'ai pas connu personnellement le temps où dans son enseignement R. LABAT abordait ce genre de textes, repaires d'idéogrammes pour lesquels la première mouture de son célèbre *Manuel* proposait d'ailleurs de précieuses listes, mais il avait déjà donné de bonnes contributions dans le domaine de la médecine et de la pharmacologie proche-orientales anciennes Il avait ainsi déjà publié sa grande œuvre, le *Traité akkadien de diagnostics et de pronostics médicaux* (1956) et il avait donné plusieurs contributions intéressantes à diverses encyclopédies, comme l'*Histoire générale des Sciences* (1957) ou le *Reallexikon der Assyriologie*, pour lequel il avait rédigé des articles comme Fehlgeburt, Fieber (1957) et Husten (1975).

C'est en souvenir de cet enseignement si novateur exercé au Collège de France, tout comme à l'École Pratique des Hautes Études, et qui demande non seulement des compétences de philologue averti mais aussi une « expérience de la pratique » que j'ai accueilli avec beaucoup de sympathie et de reconnaissance le projet d'Annie Attia et de Gilles Buisson concernant la médecine mésopotamienne et que je me suis associé à leurs efforts pour créer un lieu où soient abordés de tels sujets. Ils avaient déjà lancé à l'image de NABU le *Journal des médecines cunéiformes* (JMC), revue spécialisée dans l'accueil de recherches sur la médecine; ils étaient demandeurs, de plus, de faire venir à Paris dans le cadre d'un colloque ceux qui représentent certainement à l'heure actuelle les meilleurs spécialistes de ces textes difficiles mais essentiels pour l'histoire de la science. Le

Collège de France se trouvait donc le lieu naturel pour accueillir une telle entreprise. Je me réjouis aujourd'hui qu'ils aient persisté dans leurs efforts jusqu'à publier dans ce volume les Actes de ce colloque si stimulant à écouter.

La prochaine RAI (LVe) qui doit se tenir également au Collège de France, comme toutes les manifestations de ce genre qui l'ont précédée en France, à l'exception notoire de Strasbourg, doit voir encore un Atelier consacré à l'étude de la médecine proche-orientale. La revue JMC compte déjà 13 fascicules de parus avec de très importantes contributions (et je me réjouis qu'y soient parus des textes de Mari qui complètent l'information donnée en son temps par ARM XXVI/1). Le prochain est en bonne voie. On peut dire que c'est désormais « une affaire qui marche », et bien.

ABBREVIATIONS

A — Siglum of tablets in the collections of the Oriental Institute, University of Chicago.

A Scientific Humanist
: See Studies Sachs.

AASOR — *The Annual of the American School(s) of Oriental Research (in Jerusalem).*

AB — Assyriologische Bibliothek (Leipzig: Hinrichs).

AbB — Altbabylonische Briefe in Umschrift und Übersetzung (Leiden: Brill).
AbB 1 = F.R. Kraus, *Briefe aus dem British Museum (CT 43 und 44)*, 1964.
AbB 2 = R. Frankena, *Briefe aus dem British Museum (LIH und CT 2–33)*, 1966.
AbB 3 = R. Frankena, *Briefe aus der Leidener Sammlung (TLB IV)*, 1968.
AbB 4 = F.R. Kraus, *Briefe aus dem Archive des Šamaš-ḫāzir in Paris und Oxford (TCL 7 und OECT 3)*, 1968.
AbB 6 = R. Frankena, *Briefe aus dem Berliner Museum*, 1974.
AbB 8 = L. Cagni, *Briefe aus dem Iraq Museum (TIM II)*, 1980.
AbB 10 = F.R. Kraus, *Briefe aus kleineren westeuropäischen Sammlungen*, 1985.
AbB 11 = M. Stol, *Letters from Collections in Philadelphia, Chicago and Berkeley*, 1986.
AbB 13 = W.H. van Soldt, *Letters in the British Museum. Part 2*, 1994.
AbB 14 = K.R. Veenhof, *Letters in the Louvre*, 2005.

ABL — R.F. Harper, and L. Waterman, *Assyrian and Babylonian Letters Belonging to the Kouyunjik Collection of the British Museum*, 14 vols. (Chicago: University of Chicago Press, 1892–1914).

ABRT — J.A. Craig *Assyrian and Babylonian Religious Texts*, 2 vols., Assyriologische Bibliothek 13 (Leipzig: Hinrichs, 1895–1897).

ACh (2. Supp./Second Suppl.)
: Ch. Virolleaud, *L'astrologie chaldéenne: le livre intitulé Enuma Anu Enlil*, 5 vols., (Paris: Paul Geuthner, 1905–1912).
2.Supp. = Second Supplément.

ADFU — Ausgrabungen der deutschen Forschungsgemeinschaft in Uruk-Warka.

Adoption in Nippur
: E.C. Stone and D.I. Owen, *Adoption in Old Babylonian Nippur and the Archive of Mannum-mešu-lissur*, Mesopotamian Civilisations 3 (Winona Lake, IN: Eisenbrauns, 1990).

AEM I/1 — J.-M. Durand, *Archives Épistolaires de Mari I/1*, Archives Royales de Mari 26/1 (Paris: Editions Recherche sur les Civilisations 1988).

AEM I/2 — D. Charpin, F. Joannès, S. Lackenbaker et B. Lafont, *Archives Épistolaires de Mari* I/2, Archives Royales de Mari 26/2 (Paris: Éditions Recherche sur les Civilisations 1988).

AfO — *Archiv für Orientforschung.*

AfO Beih. — Archiv für Orientforschung, Beiheft (Berlin: Im Selbstverlage des Herausgebers; Wien: Institut für Orientalistik der Universität).

AHw	W. Von Soden, *Akkadisches Handwörterbuch*, 3 vols. (Wiesbaden: Otto Harrassowitz, 1965–1981).
Ai	Lexical series *Ana ittišu* (in MSL 1).
AIPHOS	*Annuaire de l'Institut de Philologie et d'Histoire Orientales et Slaves.*
Akk.	Akkadian
AKT	E. Bilgiç and C. Günbattı, *Ankaraner Kültepe-Texte III: Texte der Grabungskampagne 1970*, Freiburger Altorientalische Studien, Beiheft 3 (Stuttgart: Franz Steiner Verlag, 1995).
AMD	Ancient Magic and Divination (Leiden/Boston: Brill – Styx).
AMT	R. Campbell Thompson, *Assyrian Medical Texts* (London/Oxford: Clarendon Press, 1923).
AnOr	*Analecta Orientalia.*
AO	Siglum of tablets in the Louvre, (Antiquités orientales), Paris.
AOAT	Alter Orient und Altes Testament (Kevelaer/Neukirchen-Vluyn; Münster: Ugarit-Verlag).
ARM	Archives Royales de Mari (Paris: Edition Recherche sur les Civilisations). ARM 1 = G. Dossin, *Correspondance de Šamši-Addu et de ses fils*, 1950. ARM 2 = Ch. Jean, *Lettres diverses: transcrites et traduites*, 1950. ARM 3 = J.R. Kupper, *Correspondance de Kibri-Dagan; gouverneur de Terqa*, 1950. ARM 26/1 = J.-M. Durand, *Archives Épistolaires de Mari I/1*, 1988. ARM 26/2 = D. Charpin, F. Joannès, S. Lackenbaker et B. Lafont, *Archives Épistolaires de Mari* I/2, 1988.
ArOr	*Archiv Orientální.*
AS	Assyriological Studies (Oriental Institute: University of Chicago).
Augenleiden	J.C. Fincke, *Augenleiden nach keilschriftlichen Quellen. Untersuchungen zur altorientalischen Medizin*, Würzburger Medizinhistorische Forschungen 70 (Wuerzburg: Königshausen & Neumann, 2000).
AUWE	Ausgrabungen in Uruk-Warka. Endberichte (Mainz: Phillipp von Zabern).
BaF / BaghF	Baghdader Forschungen (Mainz: Philipp von Zabern).
BAK	H. Hunger, *Babylonische und assyrische Kolophone*, Alter Orient und Altes Testament 2 (Neukirchen-Vluyn: Verlag Butzon & Bercker, 1968).
BAM	F. Köcher, *Die babylonisch-assyrische Medizin in Texten und Untersuchungen* (Berlin/New York: Walter de Gruyter). BAM I–VI = F. Köcher, 1963–1980. BAM VII = M.J. Geller, *Renal and Rectal Disease Texts*, Die babylonisch-assyrische Medizin in Texten und Untersuchungen VII, 2005.
BaM – Baghd. Mitt.	*Baghdader Mitteilungen.*
BaM Beiheft	*Baghdader Mitteilungen, Beiheft.*
BARIS	British Archaeological Reports International Series (Oxford: John and Erika Hedge Ltd).
BE	The Babylonian Expedition of the University of Pennsylvania. Series A: Cuneiform Texts (Philadelphia: University of Michigan Library). BE 17 = H. Radau, *Letters to Cassite kings from the Temple Archives of Nippur* (1908).
BiOr	*Bibliotheca Orientalis.*
Birth	M. Stol, *Birth in Babylonia and the Bible: Its Mediterranean Setting*, Cuneiform Monographs 14 (Groningen: Styx Publications, 2000).
BM	Tablets in the British Museum, London.

BSOAS	*Bulletin of the School of Oriental and African Studies.*
BWL	W.G. Lambert, *Babylonian Wisdom Literature*, (Oxford: Clarendon Press, 1960).
c.	chapitre.
CAD	A.L. Oppenheim et al. eds., *The Assyrian Dictionary of the Oriental Institute of the University of Chicago* vols. 1–21 (Chicago: J.J. Augustin Verlagsbuchhandlung, Glückstadt; Winona Lake, IN: Eisenbrauns, 1956-).
CANE	*Civilizations of the Ancient Near East*, eds. J.M. Sasson and al. (New York: Scribner, 1995; 2nd edition New York: Hendrikson Publisher, 2000).
CBS	Tablets in the University Museum in Philadelphia (Catalogue of the Babylonian Section).
cf.	compare (*confer*).
CM	Cuneiform Monographs (Leiden/Boston: Brill).
CNI Publication	Carsten Niebuhr Institute Publications (Copenhagen: Carsten Niebuhr Institute Publications).
Codex Hammurapi	Law code of King Hammurapi. For edition see: M.T. Roth with a contribution by H.A. Hoffner, *Law Collections from Mesopotamia and Asia Minor*, SBL Writings from the Ancient World 6 (Atlanta: Scholars Press, 1995; 2nd ed. 1997; corr. reprint 2000).
col(s).	column(s), colonne(s).
CRRAI	Compte rendu de la Rencontre Assyriologique lnternationale.
CT	Cuneiform Texts from Babylonian Tablets in the British Museum, 54 Vols. (London: British Museum Publications, 1896-).
CTH	E. Laroche, *Catalogue des textes hittites* (Paris 1966, repr. 1971); premier supplément, 1972.
CTN	Cuneiform Texts from Nimrud (London: British School of Archaeology in Iraq).
Di	Siglum of tablets from Tell ed-Der (Belgian excavations).
Diagnostic Handbook	see TDP.
Diagnostik	N.P. Heeßel, *Babylonisch-assyrische Diagnostik*, Alter Orient und Altes Testament 43 (Munster: Ugarit-Verlag, 2000).
Dreams	A.L. Oppenheim, *The Interpretation of Dreams in the Ancient Near East. With a Translation of an Assyrian Dream-Book*, Transactions of the American Philosophical Society 46 (Philadelphia: American Philosophical Society, 1956).
e.g.	for example (*exempli gratia*).
EAE	*Enūma Anu Enlil* (Babylonian astronomical series).
ed./eds	editor(s).
Shemshara	J. Eidem and J. Laessøe, *The Shemshara Archives Vol. 1: The Letters*, Historisk-filosofiske Skrifter 23 (Copenhagen: The Royal Danish Academy of Sciences and Letters, 2001).
Emar	D. Arnaud, *Recherches au pays d'Aštata; Textes de la bibliothèque, transcriptions et traductions*, Emar 6/1–4 (Paris: Editions Recherche sur les Civilisations, 1986).
Epilepsy	M. Stol, *Epilepsy in Babylonia* (Groningen: Styx Publications, 1993).
esp.	especially.
ETCSL	The Electronic Text Corpus of Sumerian Literature, http://etcsl.orinst.ox.ac.uk/

f(f).	following (few).
FAOS (Bh.)	Freiburger Altorientalische Studien (Beihefte).
FM	*Florilegium Marianum*, Publications in the Series *Mémoires de N.A.B.U*, (Paris: SEPOA).
fn.	footnote.
FS Lambert	See Studies Lambert.
FS Sachs	See Studies Sachs.
GAG	W. von Soden, "Grundriss der Akkadischen Grammatik," *Analecta Orientalia* 33 (1995).
Gilg.	Epic of Gilgamesh. For edition see A.R. George, *The Babylonian Gilgamesh Epic* (Oxford: Oxford University Press, 2003).
HMA	R. Labat, *Hémérologies et Ménologies d'Assur* (Paris: Librairie d'Amérique et d'Orient, Adrien Maisonneuve, 1939).
HS	Siglum of tablets in the Hilprecht collection, Jena.
HSMM	Harvard Semitic Museum Monographs (Atlanta: Scholars Press).
i.e.	that is (*id est*).
IM	Siglum of tablets in the Iraq Museum, Baghdad.
In Ni.	Siglum of tablets in the Archaeological Museum, Istanbul (Nippur).
JCS	*Journal of Cuneiform Studies.*
JEOL	*Jaarbericht van het Voor-Asiatisch-Egyptisch-Genootschap Ex Oriente Lux.*
JESHO	*Journal of the Economic and Social History of the Orient.*
JMC	*Le Journal des Médecines Cunéiformes.*
JNES	*Journal of Near Eastern Studies.*
K.	Siglum of tablets in the Kuyunjik collection of the British Museum.
KADP	F. Köcher, *Keilschrifttexte zur assyrisch-babylonischen Drogen- und Pflanzenkunde* (Berlin: Akademie-Verlag, 1955).
KAR	E. Ebeling, *Keilschrifttexte aus Assur religiösen Inhalts*, Wissenschaftliche Veröffentlichungen der Deutschen Orient-Gesellschaft 28 and 34 (Leipzig: J.C. Hinrichs'sche Buchhandlung, 1915–1923).
KBo	*Keilschrifttexte aus Boghazköi*, Wissenschaftliche Veröffentlichungen der Deutschen Orient-Gesellschaft, (Leipzig/Berlin: J.C. Hinrichs'sche Buchhandlung, 1916-).
KUB	*Keilschrifturkunden aus Boghazköi* (Berlin: Akademie-Verlag). KUB IV = Ernst Weidner, 1922. KUB XXXVI = H. Otten, *Vorwiegend Mythen, Epen, Gebete und Texte in althethitischer Sprache*, 1955. KUB XXXVII = Franz Köcher, *Literarische Texte in akkadischer Sprache*, 1953.
LAPO	Littératures anciennes du Proche-Orient (Paris: éditions du Cerf). LAPO 16 = J.M. Durand, *Les documents épistolaires du palais de Mari* I, 1997. LAPO 17 = J.M. Durand, *Les documents épistolaires du palais de Mari* II, 1998. LAPO 18 = J.M. Durand, *Les documents épistolaires du palais de Mari* III, 2000.
LAS	S. Parpola, *Letters from Assyrian Scholars to the Kings Esarhaddon and Assurbanipal*, Alter Orient und Altes Testament 5, 2 vols. (Kevelaer: Butzon & Bercker, 1970–1983; repr. Winona Lake, IN: Eisenbrauns, 2007).
Li	Œuvres complètes d'Hippocrate, traduction nouvelle avec le texte grec en regard, collationné sur les manuscrits et toutes les éditions, accompagnée

d'une introduction, de commentaires médicaux, de variantes et de notes philologiques, suivie d'une table générale des matières, par Emile Littré, Adolf M. Hakkert (Amsterdam, 1961–1962; réimpression anastatique de l'édition de Paris, 1839–1861).

lit. literally.

LKA E. Ebeling, *Literarische Keilschrifttexte aus Assur* (Berlin: Akademie-Verlag, 1953).

LKU A. Falkenstein, *Literarische Keilschrifttexte aus Uruk* (Berlin: Georg Olms, 1931).

Ludlul *Ludlul bēl nēmeqi*, "I will praise the lord of wisdom". (Babylonian literary composition; for *editio princeps* see BWL).

M. Siglum of tablets found at Mari.

Magic and Rationality
Magic and Rationality in Ancient Near Eastern and Graeco-Roman Medicine, eds. H.F.R. Horstmannshoff and M. Stol in collaboration with C.R. van Tilburg, Studies in Ancient Medicine 27 (Leiden/Boston: Brill, 2004)

Magico-Medical Means
JA. Scurlock, *Magico-Medical Means of Treating Ghost-Induced Illnesses in Ancient Mesopotamia*, Ancient Magic and Divination 3 (Leiden/Boston: Brill-Styx, 2006).

MAOG *Mitteilungen der Altorientalischen Gesellschaft.*

MC Mesopotamian Civilizations (Winona Lake, IN: Eisenbrauns).

MDP R. Labat avec la collaboration de D.O. Edzard, *Textes littéraires de Suse*, Mémoires de la Délégation Archéologique en Iran 57. Mission de Susiane. Suse Ville Royale 11 (Paris: Librairie Orientaliste Paul Geuthner, 1974).

Médecine et médecins
Médecine et médecins au Proche-Orient ancien, Actes du Colloque International organisé à Lyon les 8 et 9 novembre 2002, Maison de l'Orient et de la Méditerranée eds. L. Battini and P. Villard, BAR international series 1528 (Oxford: John and Erika Hedge Ltd, 2006).

Mélanges Finet
Reflets des deux fleuves: Volume de mélanges offerts à André Finet, eds. M. Lebeau and Ph. Talon, Akkadica Supplementa 6 (Leuven: Peeters Publishers, 1989).

Mélanges Lambert
See Studies Lambert.

Memoriae Igor M. Diakonoff
Memoriae Igor M. Diakonoff; Babel und Bibel 2: Annual of Ancient Near Eastern, Old Testament, and Semitic Studies, eds. L. Kogan et al., Orientalia et Classica, Papers of the Institute of Oriental and Classical Studies 8 (Winona Lake, IN: Eisenbrauns 2005).

Mésopotamie et Elam = CRRAI 36
Mésopotamie et Elam. Actes de la XXXVIe R.A.I. Gand 10–14 juillet 1989, MHE Occasional Publications 1 (Ghent: University of Ghent, 1991).

MHE Mesopotamian History and Environment; Series 1 = *NAPR*, Series 2 = *MHEM* ; Series 3= *MHET* (Ghent: University of Ghent).

MHE, Memoirs
Mesopotamian History and Environment. (Ghent: University of Ghent).

ms(s). manuscript(s).

MSL B. Landsberger, M. Civil, et al. eds., Materialien zum sumerischen Lexikon. (Roma: Pontificium Institutum Biblicum).
MSL I = B. Landsberger, *Die Serie ana ittišu*, 1937.
MSL II = B. Landsberger, *Die Serie* Ur-e-a = *nâqu*, 1951.
MSL V = B. Landsberger, *The series* Ḫar-ra = *ḫubullu, Tablet I–IV*, 1957.
MSL IX = B. Landsberger and M. Civil, *The series* Ḫar-ra = *ḫubullu, Tablets XV*, 1967.

N.A.B.U *Nouvelles Assyriologiques Brèves et Utilitaires.*

Ni Siglum of tablets in the Archaeological Museum, Istanbul (Nippur).

no(s). number(s).

OB Old Babylonian.

OBO Orbis Biblicus et Orientalis (Freiburg/Göttingen: Vandenhoeck & Ruprecht).

OBTIV *S. Greengus, Old Babylonian Tablets from Ishchali and Vicinity*, Uitgaven van het Nederlands Historisch-Archaeologisch Instituut te Istanbul 44 (Istanbul: Nederlands Historisch-Archaeologisch Instituut / Leiden: Nederlands Instituut voor het Nabije Oosten, 1979).

obv. obverse.

OLZ *Orientalistische Literaturzeitung.*

OPSNKF Occasional Publications of the Samuel Noah Kramer Fund (Philadelphia: Babylonian Section, University Museum).

Or NS / Orientalia
Orientalia Nova Series.

OrAnt *Oriens Antiquus.*

PBS University of Pennsylvania, Publications of the Babylonian Section (Philadelphia: University Museum).
PBS 5 = A. Poebel, *Historical and Grammatical Texts*, 1914.
PBS 1/2 = H.F. Lutz, F. Henry, *Selected Sumerian and Babylonian Texts*, 1919.

Pl(s). Plate(s).

PSD Å.W. Sjöberg et. al., *The Sumerian Dictionary of the University Museum of the University of Pennsylvania* (Philadelphia: University of Pennsylvania press 1984ff.)

RA / Revue d'Assyriologie
Revue d'Assyriologie et d'Archéologie Orientale.

Renal and Rectal Disease Texts
see BAM VII.

ref(s). reference(s).

rev. reverse.

RIMA The Royal Inscriptions of Mesopotamia, Assyrian Periods (Toronto/Buffalo/London: University of Toronto Press, 1987-).
RIMA 3 = A.K. Grayson, *Assyrian Rulers of the Early First Millennium* B.C.: *II (858–745* B.C.*)*, 1996.

Rimah S. Dalley, C.B.F. Walker and J.D. Hawkins, *The Old Babylonian Tablets from Tell al Rimah* (London: British School of Archeology in Iraq, 1976).

RlA / Reallexikon der Assyriologie
E. Ebeling, et al., *Reallexikon der Assyriologie und Vorderasiatischen Archäologie* (Berlin/New York: Walter de Gruyter, 1928-).

RSO *Rivista degli Studi Orientali.*
In RSO 32: R. Labat, « Remèdes assyriens contre les affections de l'oreille, d'après un inédit du Louvre (AO, 6774) », *Rivista degli Studi Orientali* 32 (1957).

s.v. under the entry (*sub voce*).

SAA State Archives of Assyria (Helsinki: The Neo-Assyrian Text Corpus Project).
SAA 2 = S. Parpola and K. Watanabe, *Neo-Assyrian Treaties and Loyalty Oath*, 1988.
SAA 4 = I. Starr, *Queries to the Sungod: Divination and Politics*, 1990.
SAA 8 = H. Hunger, *Astrological Reports to Assyrian Kings*, 1992.
SAA 10 = S. Parpola, *Letters from Assyrian and Babylonian Scholars*, 1993.

SAAS State Archives of Assyria Studies (Helsinki: The Neo-Assyrian Text Corpus Project).

SA.GIG diagnostic series, see: Diagnostik and Diagnostic Handbook.

Sin and Sanction
Sin and Sanction in Israel and Mesopotamia – a comparative study, Studia Semitica Neerlandica 22 (Assen/Maastricht: van Gorcum, 1985).

SLB W. Leemans, *Legal and Administrative Documents of the Time of Hammurabi and Samsuiluna (Mainly from Lagaba)* Studia ad tabulas cuneiformes collectas a F.M. Th. de Liagre Bohl pertinentia (Leiden: Brill, 1960).

SpTU / SpBTU
Spätbabylonische Texte aus Uruk (Berlin: Gebr. Mann).
I: H. Hunger, *Spätbabylonische Texte aus Uruk*, I, Ausgrabungen der Deutschen Forschungsgemeinschaft in Uruk-Warka 10, 1976.
II: E. von Weiher, *Spätbabylonische Texte aus Uruk*, II, Ausgrabungen der Deutschen Forschungsgemeinschaft in Uruk-Warka 10, 1983.
IV: E. von Weiher, *Spätbabylonische Texte aus dem Planquadrat U 18*, Ausgrabungen in Uruk-Warka. Endberichte 12, 1993.
V: E. von Weiher, *Spätbabylonische Texte aus dem Planquadrat U 18*, Ausgrabungen in Uruk-Warka. Endberichte 13, 1998.

StBoT Studien zu den Bogazköy-Texten (Wiesbaden: Harrassowitz).

STT *The Sultantepe Tablets* (London/Bradford: Percy Lund, Humphries and Company Ltd.
STT I = O.R. Gurney and J.J. Finkelstein, *The Sultantepe Tablets* I, 1957
STT II = O.R. Gurney and P. Hulin, *The Sultantepe Tablets* II, 1964.

Studies Fronzaroli
Semitic and Assyriological Studies Presented to Pelio Fronzaroli by Pupils and Colleagues, ed. P. Marrassini (Wiesbaden: Harrassowitz Verlag, 2003).

Studies Lambert
Wisdom, Gods and Literature. Studies in Assyriology in Honour of W.G. Lambert, eds. A.R. George and I.L. Finkel, (Winona Lake, IN: Eisenbrauns, 2000).

Studies Landsberger
Studies in Honor of Benno Landsberger on his Seventy-Fifth Birthday, April 21, 1965, eds. H.G. Güterbock and T. Jacobsen, Assyriological Studies 16 (Chicago Oriental Institute: University of Chicago, 1965).

Studies Leichty
If a Man Builds a Joyful House: Assyriological Studies in Honor of Erle Verdun Leichty, eds. A.K. Guinan, M. de J. Ellis, A.J. Ferrara, Cuneiform Monographs 31 (Leiden/London: Brill, 2006).

Studies Sachs
: *A Scientific Humanist: Studies in Memory of Abraham Sachs*, eds. E. Leichty, M. de J. Ellis, and P. Gerardi, Occasional Publications of the Samuel Noah Kramer Fund 9 (Philadelphia: The University Museum, 1988)

Studies Sjöberg
: *DUMU-E$_2$-DUB-BA-A: Studies in Honor of Å. W. Sjöberg*, eds. H. Behrens, D. Loding and M. Roth, Occasional Publications of the Samuel Noah Kramer Fund 11 (Philadelphia: Babylonian Section, University Museum, 1989).

s.v. under the entry (*sub voce*).

Šurpu Series of incantations. The most recent edition is: E. Reiner, *Šurpu: A Collection of Sumerian and Akkadian Incantations*, Archiv für Orientforschung, Beiheft 11 (Wien: Institut für Orientalistik der Universität, 1958).

t. tome.

TBP F.R. Kraus, *Texte zur babylonischen Physiognomatik*, Archiv für Orientforschung 3 (Berlin: Im Selbstverlage des Herausgebers, 1939).

TCS Texts from Cuneiform Sources (New York: J.J. Augustin).

TdH Texte der Hethiter (Heidelberg: Universitätsverlag C. Winter).

TDP R. Labat, *Traité akkadien de diagnostics et pronostics médicaux I–II* (Paris: Académie Internationale d'Histoire des Sciences, 1951). Note: Tablets 15–33 newly edited by Heeßel, *Diagnostik*.

TH Siglum of tablets in the British Museum.

TIM Texts in the Iraq Museum.
TIM I = A. Al-Zeebari *Old Babylonian Letters* (Baghdad: Dar Al-Jumbari Press, 1964).
TIM II = J. Van Dijk, *Cuneiform Texts: Old Babylonian Letters and related Material* (Wiesbaden: Harrassowitz, 1965).

TMHC NF Texte und Materialien der Frau Professor Hilprecht Collection of Babylonian Antiquities im Eigentum der Universität Jena, Neue Folge.

UCP University of California Publications in Semitic Philology (Berkeley: University of California Press).
UCP 9 = H.F. Lutz, *Neo-Babylonian Administrative Documents from Erech*, 1927.

UET Ur Excavations, Texts (London: Oxford University Press for The Trustees of the two Museums).
UET 3 = Léon Legrain, *Business Documents of the third Dynasty of Ur*, 1937.
UET 5 = H.H. Figulla and W.J. Martin, *Letters and Documents of the Old-Babylonian Period*, 1953.

UF Ugarit-Forschungen (Kevelaer/Neukirchen-Vluyn).

Ugaritica / Ug
: Ugaritica. Mission de Ras Shamra (Paris: Editions Recherche sur les Civilisations, 1939–1978)

UGU Medical series *šumma amēlu muḫḫašu umma ukāl*. Tablet 1 edited by M. Worthington in *JMC* 5 (2005); Tablet 2 edited by A. Attia and G. Buisson in *JMC* 1 (2003).

Uh lexical series, Urra-hubullu, see MSL V.

UM Tablet siglum of the University Museum, Philadelphia

Ur-Namma lawcode
Law code. For edition see: M.T. Roth with a contribution by H.A. Hoffner, *Law Collections from Mesopotamia and Asia Minor* SBL Writings from the Ancient World 6 (Atlanta: Scholars Press, 1995; 2nd ed. 1997; corr. reprint 2000).

VAT Siglum of tablets in the Vorderasiatisches Museum, Berlin.

vs. versus.

W. Field numbers of tablets excavated at Uruk/Warka.

WVDOG Wissenschaftliche Veröffentlichungen der Deutschen Orient-Gesellschaft (Leipzig: J.C. Hinrichs'sche Buchhandlung).

ZA / Zeitschrift für Assyriologie
until 1938: *Zeitschrift für Assyriologie und verwandte Gebiete*; from 1939: *Zeitschrift für Assyriologie und Vorderasiatische Archäologie* (Leipzig; Berlin 1886-).

LIST OF CONTRIBUTORS

BARBARA BÖCK, Ph.D. (1996) in Assyriology, Freie Universität Berlin, is tenured scientist at the CSIC in Madrid. She has published on scholarly texts from first millennium Mesopotamia, in particular on divination, magic, and medicine. Her works include: *Die babylonisch-assyrische Morphoskopie* (Wien 2000) and *Das Handbuch Muššu'u "Einreibung". Eine Serie sumerischer und akkadischer Beschwörungen aus dem 1. Jt. v.Chr.* (Madrid 2007).

PAUL DEMONT is professor of Greek at Paris-Sorbonne University and has published extensively on ancient humoral medicine and its transmission in modern times. His work includes: *La cité grecque archaïque et classique et l'idéal de tranquillité* (Paris 1990).

JEANETTE C. FINCKE, Ph.D. (1999) in Assyriology, Julius-Maximilians-Universität Würzburg, Germany, is researcher at Leiden University. She has published on cuneiform medicine, divination in Mesopotamia and the Hittite kingdom as well as on the cuneiform tablets from the Assyrian capital Nineveh written in Babylonian ductus.

NILS. P. HEEßEL, Ph.D. (1999) in Assyriology, University of Heidelberg, is research assistant at Heidelberg Academy of Sciences. He published on Ancient Near East Medicine, Divination, and History of Religion. He is the author of *Divinatorische Texte I, Keilschrifttexte aus Assur literarischen Inhalts 1* (Wiesbaden 2007).

MARTEN STOL, Ph.D. in Assyriology (1976), Leiden University, is professor emeritus of Assyriology at the Vrije Universiteit, Amsterdam. He publishes on the Old Babylonian period and the Babylonian medical texts. One of his latest books is *Birth in Babylonia and the Bible* (STYX-Brill, 2000).

MARTIN WORTHINGTON, Ph.D. (2007) in Assyriology, University of Cambridge, is a research fellow at St John's College, Cambridge. His research interests include Mesopotamian medicine, magic, and literature, and Akkadian grammar.

INTRODUCTION
"OEIL MALADE ET MAUVAIS OEIL"

Markham J. Geller

The present group of papers resulted from a colloquium at the Collège de France in June 2006, on the theme of "oeil malade et mauvais oeil" (the sick eye and the evil eye), intending to highlight both the magical and medical aspects of ancient medicine. The papers all address some of the most important issues within ancient Babylonian and Greek medicine from different perspectives. Some papers discuss the social aspects of healing, trying to determine who the healers were and in what context they operated, while other authors examine the technical aspects of therapy, such as the type of plants used and how they were treated. As with every new publication, it is a good idea to assess what progress has been made in understanding ancient medicine, even if our assessment is likely to be provisional, since it is easy to lose sight of the general picture when concentrating upon the essential details and data.

There are three elusive and rather thorny themes to bear in mind while evaluating the present collection of papers and the information presented in them. The themes are basic ones and concern 1) comparisons between Babylonian medicine and other contemporary systems of medicine in the region 2) the relationship(s) between magic and medicine, and 3) the social role of medicine/therapy within Babylonian society.

What we have from Mesopotamia, however, is an extremely valuable and large corpus of medicine which needs to be edited, translated, and explicated, as well as exploring any connections with other systems of medicine in the Ancient Near East. Egyptian medicine is certainly one candidate for comparison, since Egypt has its own corpus of medical texts, most of which are, however, much earlier than those in Akkadian, dating from an era corresponding to the Old Babylonian period in Mesopotamia, when medical texts are only sparsely attested. Nevertheless, Egyptian medicine contains much in the way of therapeutic texts and recipes, although we find nothing in the way of prognosis or diagnosic texts comparable to the Babylonian Diagnostic Handbook.

Furthermore, Egyptian texts dating from the second millennium B.C. have no late copies indicating that they were transmitted and studied in later periods, either in oral or written form. This makes precise textual comparisons between Akkadian and Egyptian medical texts problematic, since we would ideally prefer to compare texts from the same period.

With Greek medicine, however, the situation is much more promising, since much of Akkadian medicine from the latter first millennium B.C. has contemporaneous Greek counterparts showing many similar features. The Hippocratic corpus, in particular, has examples of prognosis and proverbial medical literature which look very much like Akkadian medicine, and there is a certain amount of therapeutic literature from this same corpus which also resembles Akkadian recipes. Paul Demont's article ends on this very note, citing examples of texts from the Hippocratic treatise *Diseases II*, which is known to come from an early stratum of the Hippocratic corpus, and these texts look remarkably similar to what we find in Akkadian, although these comparisons have never been studied systematically.

The complex relationship between magic and medicine is arguably better attested in Mesopotamia than in most other ancient sources, judging by the sheer quantity and variety of both incantations and medical texts which the cuneiform tablets have to offer. The relationships between magic and medicine in Mesopotamia are both complex and subtle, since the configuration of therapeutic practices is divided between magic and medicine, divination, exorcism and recipe-based treatment, with an extensive literature in all genres of texts.

The roles of the two main healing professionals, the *āšipu* and *asû*, sufficiently overlap to prevent a clear determination of their respective roles. Within the royal court, for instance, both the exorcist and *asû* appear to offer similar treatments, as pointed out by Barbara Böck in the present volume. The *āšipu*-exorcist appears to have a good deal of medical knowledge and in fact is responsible for prognosis and diagnosis (which to us would appear counter-intuitive), while the *asû* was equally responsible for copying incantations into his medical recipes. Furthermore, we have no idea about the training of such personnel, a point which Geoffrey Lloyd takes up in reference to ancient Greek and Chinese physicians. He points out that:

> None had legally recognized qualifications, such as exist for modern biomedical practitioners, who receive licenses to practise only after they have finished thier training in approved medical schools. But they had clearly

> defined roles in treating the sick and were marked out from other lay people by their – supposed – greater knowledge and skill, certainly their greater experience in the matter. Second in both ancient societies [Greece and China] some such specialists at least (not all) moved away from any assumption that sickness was brought about by spirits or demonic forces or could be cured by prayer or ritual alone.[1]

Lloyd's point is a controversial one, since Greek treatises on medicine regularly omit to mention belief in divine interference in human affairs, and especially ill-health. Just as in Greece there is no obligatory contradiction between belief in gods and medical theory, there is also within Mesopotamia no clear-cut division between exorcist and doctor, with one relying upon incantations and rituals while the other relies upon drugs and recipes. One marked difference between the Babylonian *āšipu* and *asû*, of course, is that the former is a priest while the latter was a layman, and the distinction is socially very important. The *āšipu* enjoyed all the privileges of the temple, both its prestige and wealth, while the latter was not even allowed entry to the temple precincts, which was restricted to the *ēreb bīti*, "one permitted to enter to temple", a common term for a priest. The *asû* was essentially a peddler of drugs, although we have little information about how he earned his livelihood (see below). There is no specific Akkadian term for "surgeon" as a professional title (which applies to Greece as well).

One intriguing question, which so far has not been asked, is whether either of these terms, *āšipu* or *asû*, conforms to Greek *iatros* or "doctor". In his comprehensive article in this volume, Paul Demont refers to the Mycenean term *i-a-te* (= *iatros*) from a Pylos tablet from 1200 B.C., allowing for plenty of opportunity to connect this term with an Akkadian equivalent. In the Iliad, this same word for doctor applied to two sons of Asclepius who were famous for extracting arrows and for soothing drugs.[2] What Akkadian term would correspond? We have no reports from battles or military doctors from Mesopotamia, nor is it likely that either Akkadian professional title corresponds to *iatros*. This may be the reason why Herodotus himself was puzzled when he allegedly visited Babylon, as Martin Worthington notes in his article below, and why Herodotus reported that Babylonians have no use for physicians but

[1] G.E.R. Lloyd, *Cognitive Variations* (Oxford: Oxford University Press, 2007), 89.

[2] G.E.R. Lloyd, *In the Grip of Disease. Studies in the Greek Imagination* (Oxford: Oxford University Press, 2003), 17.

simply carry the patients into the market place and seek advice from anyone passing by; Herodotus also notes that anyone passing was obliged to inquire about the patient's illness.[3] The reason behind Herodotus's statement may be that he could indeed find no equivalent to the *iatros* among the Babylonian healing professionals, since the *āšipu* as exorcist was hardly appropriate and the *asû* was much more akin to the Greek root-cutter than physician.

One might conclude that the respective roles of *āšipu* and *asû* could reflect a genuine difference between magic and medicine, to the extent that, theoretically at least, magic and exorcism address themselves to the patient's mental state and anxieties, while medicine tended to concentrate on physical symptoms, such as pain, fever, and seizures. Although such a sweeping supposition might be valid in some cases (hence *oeil malade* vs. *mauvais oeil*), nevertheless there is plenty of contradictory evidence from the Akkadian medical corpus itself, for which many types of psychological distress are treated with ordinary drugs and recipes, in addition to incantations.[4] The corpus of Akkadian medical texts includes many which can be labelled as "magico-medical", in which ailments associated with witchcraft are treated with medical recipes rather than simply through Maqlû-type incantations.[5] Although there are many incantations which are clearly not medical and many therapeutic texts which are clearly not magic, the grey area of texts sharing both categories is inconvenient for scholars trying to come up with a workable typology of healing arts in Mesopotamia. A good example of this mixed genre of medicine and magic are medical texts dealing with diseases of the eyes, which are often treated with a combination of drug therapy and incantations. Here are examples from a standard collection of therapeutic texts from Nineveh dealing with eye disease:

---

[3] This particular passage in Herodotus (*Histories* I 197) has a parallel in the Odyssey (4. 230 f.), which refers to the fact that in Egypt every man is a potential healer, "wise above all men", and elsewhere in the Odyssey Homer refers to the use of an Egyptian drug (*pharmakon*), see Odyssey IV 221 and Fr. Graf, *La magie dans l'antiquité gréco-romaine* (Paris: Les Belles Lettres, 1994) translated by F. Philip, *Magic in the Ancient World* (Cambridge, MA/London: Harvard University Press, 1997), 28.

[4] See the discussion in JA. Scurlock, *Magico-Medical Means of Treating Ghost-Induced Illnesses in Ancient Mesopotamia*, Ancient Magic and Divination 3 (Leiden/Boston: Brill-Styx, 2006), 16 ff.

[5] See D. Schwemer, *Abwehrzauber und Behexung* (Wiesbaden, 2007), 165 ff.

> If a man's eyes are full of blood, daub (them) with *ashar* in ghee.
> Mix *maštakal* and *taramuš* in equal amounts, crush *nikiptu*-plant in ghee, daub his eyes.[6]

Combined with standard "medicine" such as this, we also find incantations in the same tablets:

> Incantation. The look sees, the opened eye sees, the evil eye sees evil, the opened eye sees evil. The two of them are daughters of Anu, in between whom a clay-wall is built, one sister does not go to meet her sister. Whom shall I send to the Daughers of Anu of Heaven? Let them take up their *hulūlu*-stone jars and jugs of pure green-lapis, let them draw water and *extinguish* the cloudy, dim and blurred eyes. Incantation spell.[7]

On the other hand, Jeanette Fincke's article in the present collection presents two medical texts dealing with eye disease, and although incomplete neither text shows any evidence of incantations, which may have been optional or at least were not a *de rigueur* feature of medical tablets. It is worth noting, however, that Egyptian medicine dealing with eye disease shows this same combination of drugs and incantations.[8] Examples come from Papyrus Ebers, which resemble the eye recipes in Fincke's contribution to this volume:

> Autre (remède), pour chasser le sang qui est dans les yeux : ocre crouge (*tjerou*) : 1 ; malachite : 4 ; galène : 1 ; bois pourri : 1 ; plante-*djaret* : 1 ; eau : 1. (Ce) sera broyé finement et placé dans les yeux (Eb. 348).[9]

> Autre (remède) pour chasser le sang qui est dans les yeux : deux coupes d'argile, une avec de la farine d'épeautre-*mimi* et du lait d'une femme ayant mis au monde un enfant mâle, l'autre avec du lait (de vache). (Ce) sera laissé au repos la nuit à la rosée. Tu devras remplir le matin tes yeux avec cette farine (d'épeautre). Après cela, tu devras te laver les yeux avec ce lait quatre fois par jour (Eb. 384).[10]

The latter recipe is followed immediately by an incantation:

> Autre (remède), pour chasser la montée des sérosités dans les yeux : "Viens, malachite ! Viens, malachite ! Viens, la verte ! Viens écoulement de l'oeil

6 Cf. the duplicate texts BAM 510 i 41′ // 513 i 31′ // 514 i 49′ A general feature of this text is that medical recipes appear on the obverse but much of the reverse is taken up with incantations. An edition of these tablets is scheduled to appear in a forthcoming number of *JMC*.

7 BAM 510 iii 17–21 // 513 iii 18′–22′//514 iii 22′–26′//Emar 738: 6′–8′.

8 See T. Bardinet, *Les papyrus médicaux de l'Egypte pharonique* (Paris: Fayard, 1995), 178.

9 Bardinet, *Les papyrus médicaux*, 304.

10 Bardinet, *Les papyrus médicaux*, 308.

> d'Horus ! Viens, rejet de l'oeil d'Atoum ! Viens, sécrétion sortie d'Osiris ! Viens à lui et chasse pour lui les sérosités (littéralement : 'l'eau'), le pus, le sang, ..." Paroles à réciter sur de la malachite pilée dans du miel fermenté. Il sera aussi pilé pour eux (= les yeux) du souchet comestible et (ce) sera appliqué aux yeux. Vraiment efficace. (Eb. 385).[11]

Although we generally lack the full range of magical texts from Greece that we have from Mesopotamia, this does not mean that Greeks had little use for magic within their notions of medicine.[12] Paul Demont's article below discusses the Hippocratic treatise *On the Sacred Disease*, a polemic against popular notions of magic within medicine. Demont points out, however, that the notion of "sacred disease" occurs in common parlance, such as the way Herodotus referred to Cambyses' madness as an example of a "sacred disease". The argument within this Hippocratic treatise has remained at the centre of the dispute between those who see ancient medicine in its "magical-religious" or "rational" aspects, and the debate continues.[13]

Much of the difference between magic and medicine is social rather than purely intellectual. The practitioners themselves obviously had a hand in deciding what types of therapies to use, depending upon the particular symptoms presented by the patient. Unfortunately, we know very little about the social setting of therapy, except perhaps that the exorcist appeared to have visited the patient at home, since hospitals were a later Byzantine invention, nor is there any recognised Mesopotamian equivalent to the Aesclepion of the Greco-Roman world. We know nothing about the conditions under which the patient was examined, or even by whom, and whether the patient was alone or surrounded by his family at the time. We have no details as to how the practitioner was paid, or by whom, or how the patient knew to which type of healer to turn.

Martin's Worthington's contribution to the present volume helps us somewhat in this respect, since he has gone to the trouble of seeking out relevant correspondence from among the large number of Akkadian private letters which refer in some way to the healing arts. These letters are an invaluable source for collateral information about Babylonian medicine, since they refer to physicians within the context of everyday

11 Bardinet, *Les papyrus médicaux*, 308 f.
12 See Graf *Magic*, 43 ff.
13 See Graf, *Magic*, 30 ff.

life.[14] Moreover, these letters allow us to eavesdrop on private and confidential exchanges between doctor and patient, and there is no equivalent to such correspondence within the vast corpus of Greek medicine.[15]

It would be helpful to know who actually composed medical texts and how any medical text was received or altered by colleagues and later followers. As it is, almost all medical texts are anonymous and we know virtually nothing about who composed them. This is one feature, however, which Babylonian and Greek medicine have in common, since only one treatise in the entire Hippocratic corpus, *On the Nature of Man*, is known to have been composed by Hippocrates' son-in-law Polybus,[16] while all other treatises in the corpus are likely to have been composed and revised by several unknown hands.[17]

In addition to not knowing about the physicians and scholars who composed our texts, we also know little about the patients, with the exception of the patients mentioned in the corpus of cuneiform letters, mentioned above. Thanks to Neo-Assyrian letters, we know, for example, that King Esarhaddon suffered from a debilitating chronic disease, although we do not know which recipes from our extensive medical corpus may have been prescribed for his condition. Medical texts themselves never refer to patients by name, since they are primarily concerned with disease and symptoms, rather than with patients. We have nothing from Mesopotamia equivalent to the work of the renowned Classical orator Aelius Aristides, who was also a great hypochondriac and chronicled in great detail both his symptoms and treatments.[18]

This is where Nils Heeßel's contribution to the present volume offers intriguing new data. For the very first time, we have first-hand evidence of an actual physician named Rabâ-ša-Marduk, with a well-established reputation, whose activities are attested both in Babylonia and at the Hittite royal court, where he was invited as a resident medical expert some time after 1285 B.C. At the same time, we have one example of a medical

---

[14] Neo-Assyrian letters dealing with medical problems at the Assyrian royal court have been studied in some detail by C. Jean, *La magie néo-assyrienne en contexte: recherche sur le métier d'exorciste et le concept d'*āšipūtu, State Archives of Assyria Studies 17 (Helsinki: The Neo-Assyrian Text Corpus Project, 2006).

[15] Worthington's Section 3 (Availability and affordability) provides some useful data regarding the payment of the *asû*, but these isolated examples fall far short of explaining generally how medical practitioners were paid and at what rate.

[16] According to both Aristotle and *Anonymus Londinensis*.

[17] Lloyd, *Grip*, 41 f.

[18] See V. Nutton, *Ancient Medicine* (London and New York: Routledge, 2004), 276–279.

text written in Babylonia, dealing with migraine, which contains the signature of this same physician Rabâ-ša-Marduk in the colophon of the tablet.[19] There is a chance that such an eminent physician would actually have composed this tablet rather than simply copied it as an ordinary scribe. Heeßel is understandably cautious and but does suggest that since the colophon does not refer to the tablet being copied from an previous *Vorlage*, it might represent an original composition and hence the first example of tablet bearing the name of its author. As Heeßel points out, comparison shows that this early 13th century tablet is essentially a "forerunner" of a later standard medical composition, probably due to the fact that Rabâ-ša-Marduk's tablet was confiscated with many other tablets from Babylonia and brought to Tiglath-Pileser's royal library in 1220 B.C. We will never know whether Rabâ-ša-Marduk himself composed this text or merely copied the tablet, but we can take into account some circumstantial evidence. The very fact that Rabâ-ša-Marduk was invited to the Hittite capital suggests that he was indeed an authority on medicine, rather than simply a copyist of medical tablets, and only a century later another noted scholar, Esagil-kīn-apli, was credited with the editon of medical diagnostic omens.[20] This might point to the 13th–12th centuries as the likely period during which texts were being composed and edited, as already suggested by Erica Reiner and others.[21]

Even if we could establish that the 13th century B.C. scholar/physician Rabâ-ša-Marduk was the author of an isolated medical text, this is far from providing us with other information we require about the nature of the medical corpus and how it was composed, edited, and transmitted over many generations of scribal activity. There is nothing comparable in the Babylonian world to Galen's commentary on Hippocrates and Plato,[22] or the encyclopedia of Oribasius based mostly upon Galen's work.

---

[19] BAM 11. The medical condition is known by its Sumerogram label, sag.ki.dab.ba, and Rabâ-ša-Marduk's tablet duplicates BAM 482, which is Tablet 2 of the Series *šumma amēlu muhhašu umma ukāl*, for which A. Attia and G. Buisson, « Edition de texte: 'Si le crâne d'un homme contient de la chaleur, deuxième tablette' », *Le Journal des Médecines Cunéiformes* 1 (2003): 3–24.

[20] This unique colophon was published by I.L. Finkel, "Adad-pala-iddina, Esagil-kīn-apli, and the Series SA.GIG," in *A Scientific Humanist: Studies in Memory of Abraham Sachs*, eds. E. Leichty, M. deJ. Ellis, and P. Gerardi, Occasional Publications of the Samuel Noah Kramer Fund 9 (Philadelphia: the University Museum, 1988), 1–26, 143–159.

[21] E. Reiner, *Šurpu: A Collection of Sumerian and Akkadian Incantations*, Archiv für Orientforschung, Beiheft 11 (Graz, 1958, repr. Osnabrueck: Biblio Verlag, 1970), 2.

[22] Galen, *On the Opinions of Hippocrates and Plato.*

The few medical commentaries we possess mostly provide synonyms for technical words appearing in medical texts, and these have been used to advantage by Marten Stol in his contribution in this volume.

Technical meanings of Akkadian medical terminology also raise challenging obstacles. Marten Stol's article in the present volume illustrates this very well, since even a basic expression for being ill in Akkadian needs to be subjected to thorough philological analysis. Stol has studied the Akkadian noun *sili'tu* "illness" with its cognate verb *salā'u* "to be ill", to distinguish them from another more common word *murṣu* "illness" and *marāṣu* "to be ill". The difference between these two terms has a parallel within Greek terminology, namely *nosos* and *pathe*, both words referring virtually interchangeably in Greek medicine to disease and illness. According to Lloyd, *nosos* "disease" is the antonym of *hygiea*, "health" and in addition to being a generic term of physical disease, *nosos* can also refer to madness, love-sickness, "senselessness" (*anoia*) and an "unbridled tongue".[23] *Pathe*, on the other hand, is a general term for affection and suffering, and as Lloyd points out, "when doctors deal with the *pathe* of their patients, they were dealing, potentially, with everything that happened to them, not just what they could identify as specific diseases."[24] We would suggest that the distinction between *nosos* and *pathe* parallels some of the semantic differences be Akkadian *sili'tu* and *murṣu*. As Stol explains in exemplary detail, *sili'tu* is a word specifically referring to disease in various contexts, either chronic or specific. By way of contrast, the synonym *murṣu* is a much more general term implying "illness", "trouble", "suffering", or even "annoyance", as a noun derived from a verb *marāṣu*, and in any case it has a much wider semantic range than *sili'tu*.

The problem of terminology is also taken up by Barbara Böck in her article in this volume on medical technology, explaining how plants and *materia medica* were handled in recipes in order to extract the properties necessary for the preparation of drugs. It is interesting that there is no specific Akkadian technical term for "recipe", since the word which is usually applied, *bulṭu*, is in fact a general word for "cure". There is no equivalent Akkadian term for Greek *pharmakon*, which can also apply in fact to incantations and charms as well as to poisons. It is also somewhat surprising that we have no mention of poisons within

[23] Lloyd, *Grip*, 12.

[24] Lloyd, *Grip* 12. See also M. Tecusan, *The Fragments of the Methodists. Methodism outside Soranus. Vol. 1: Text and Translation. Studies in Ancient Medicine, 24/1*. (Leiden: Brill, 2004), 10.

Akkadian medicine, as we have within Greco-Roman medicine, although there are some general comparisons with Greek pharmacology which require study. As Lloyd explains,

> The process of acquiring knowledge of drugs and poisons was haphazard and unsystematic. There was no reliable, standardized, way in which a doctor could record and pass on the information he had gained in his own clinical practice. Such knowledge was handed on largely by word of mouth, although the subject was discussed ... both by natural philosophers such as Theophrastus, and by doctors such as Dioscorides. The accounts of the effects of drugs that we have in our written sources all suffer from the indeterminacies I have mentioned, starting with the problem of identifying the plants in question, and including also vagueness in the accounts of how to collect and prepare the drug and even the lack of standardization of weights and measures. The root-cutters were often secretive and they surrounded their procedures with myths and rituals.[25]

The very same statement could be made about Babylonian pharmacology, which was equally unsystematic in how drugs were prescribed, with little exact notion of dosage and potency. Moreover, we have no knowledge of how our recipes were actually composed, and which drugs were chosen as effective against which diseases, considering the fact that no clinical trials were possible in antiquity. Martin Worthington, at the end of his contribution, shows how plants were listed in a remarkably similar order even within different types of texts, indicating that lists of medicinal plants were probably learned by heart as part of scribal training. This tells us little about how recipes themselves were concocted, if we begin with the modern assumption that each item of *materia medica* was selected because of some effective potency or effect on the body.

It is likely that Babylonians had some idea of the properties of medicinal plants and minerals, not entirely dissimilar to those known to Dioscorides.[26] Babylonians, however, were not as systematic as the Greeks in classifying plants according to their medicinal properties, such as their "warming", "astringent", or "diuretic" effects.[27] Nevertheless, similar types of procedures were followed by both Babylonian and Greek pharmacologists in preparing their drugs. Barbara Böck's description of the way Babylonian plants were dried before use closely matches Dioscorides'

---

[25] Lloyd, *Variations*, 95.

[26] More of this will be clear to us when the edition of Uruanna will be published, as promised by Barbara Böck in her footnote 3.

[27] See J. Riddle, *Dioscorides on Pharmacy and Medicine* (Austin: University of Texas Press, 1985), 33 f.

instructions for preparing the plant *daphne*: "gather the leaves at harvest time, dry them in the shade, beat them (in a mortar, assumed), but take care to remove the strings before administration."[28] Moreover, we have several important Akkadian lexical lists of plants, stones, and wounds (or sores, *simmu*), based on their *šiknu*, an Akkadian term for "character" or "nature" corresponding quite closely to Greek *phusis*, "nature", which originally referred to the nature of plants, etc., and only later developed a more general meaning referring to nature as a whole.[29] As the author of *On the Sacred Disease* himself says, "Each [disease] has a nature (*phusis*) and power (*dunamis*) of its own",[30] and it is likely that the similarity in meaning of Greek *phusis* and Akkadian *šiknu* may not be entirely coincidental.

Still, it is important to ask why Greek and Babylonian medicine do not resemble each other even more than the parallels suggested here. Considering the many inscriptions from temple medicine, such as the Asclepion, which bear witness to patients being miraculously healed through incubation and remedies being sent by dreams,[31] it remains surprising that no examples of incubation as a form of therapy have been found in a Mesopotamian context. On the other hand, there are no extant Hippocratic eye-disease recipes, for instance, which resemble the two medical tablets published by Jeanette Fincke in the present volume. Some recipes survive among the fragments of the later Greek Methodist school, but the Hippocratic corpus itself contains few examples of the kind of therapeutic texts which we know from Mesopotamia. The differences between Greek and Babylonian medicine are significant in themselves and deserve to be the subject of further study.

---

[28] Riddle, *Dioscorides*, 74. Riddle further notes (ibid.) Dioscorides's instructions for preparing cinnamon, that "it be dried in the shade after being beaten and put in wine", and similar such instructions can easily be found in Akkadian medical recipes; see Dietlinde Goltz, *Studien zur altorientalischen und griechischen Heilkunde. Therapie—Arzneibereitung - Rezeptstruktur* (Wiesbaden: Franz Steiner Verlag, 1974), 29f. Many further parallels between Babylonian medical texts and Dioscorides remained to be investigated; see for example, Riddle, *Dioscorides*, 90, giving a recipe which has been compared with Papyrus Ebers (No. 98), although Akkadian recipes are closer. See also Dioscorides' statement that copper vessels are a suitable container for eye drugs (Riddle, *Dioscorides*, 73), for which we have the copper *tamgussu*-bowl frequently used in Babylonian recipes.

[29] See Lloyd, *Variations*, 133ff.

[30] Hippocrates, *On the Sacred Disease* XXI, translation W.H. S Jones, The Loeb Classical Library 148 (Cambridge, MA./London: Harvard University Press, 1923, reprinted 1998), 182f.

[31] See E.J. Edelstein and L. Edelstein, *Asclepius: A Collection and Interpretation of the Testimonies* (Baltimore: The Johns Hopkins University Press, 1998).

Real progress in understanding Babylonian medicine will hardly come from comparisons with modern diagnosis and treatment of disease, or from trying to identify ancient with modern plants.[32] The very best we can hope for is to try to identify Akkadian diseases and plants with their Greco-Roman or even Egyptian counterparts, in trying to bring Mesopotamia into the mainstream of medical history. There is little point in circumventing the long history of medicine, from antiquity to Middle Ages to modern medicine, by attempting to identify Akkadian words with modern medical terminology. Ancient physicians had neither instruments or laboratories in which to test hypotheses, and it was often difficult to tell the difference between a genuine doctor and a quack, since neither was more or less capable of curing a patient. We can, however, try to see how Babylonian medicine faced the same challenges encountered by neighbouring systems of medicine from Egypt and Greco-Roman worlds, to see what strategies Babylonian medicine may have shared with other systems of medicine to deal with similar problems of diagnosis, prognosis, and treatment of disease.

[32] This is the methodological flaw in the work of JA. Scurlock and B.R. Andersen, *Diagnoses in Assyrian and Babylonian Medicine. Ancient Sources, Translations, and Modern Medical Analyses* (Urbana/Chicago: University of Illinois Press, 2005), since most of the comparisons with modern medicine are highly speculative and in almost every instance open to challenge. The same can be said for attempts to identify Akkadian plants with modern drugs, see L. Renault, "A Short Note on JA Scurlock's Recent Identification of the *kamantu*-Plant with *Lawsonia inermis L.*," *Le Journal des Médecines Cunéiformes* 10 (2007): 47–48.

THE BABYLONIAN PHYSICIAN RABÂ-ŠA-MARDUK. ANOTHER LOOK AT PHYSICIANS AND EXORCISTS IN THE ANCIENT NEAR EAST*

Nils P. Heeßel

When Edith Ritter published her article "Magical-Expert (=*Āšipu*) and Physician (=*Asû*). Notes on Two Complementary Professions in Babylonian Medicine" in the widely read Landsberger Festschrift in 1965,[1] the problem of the two healing professions in Ancient Mesopotamia seemed to be solved at last. Ritter argued that the two professions *āšipu* "exorcist" and *asû* "physician" could be distinguished along the lines of magic vs. medicine, irrationality vs. rationality. The *āšipu* was the magical-expert who countered disease by charms and incantations, in other words by magical means. The *asû*, by contrast, was the physician who healed the sick with bandages and poultices, by his medical craft, which was rational. This rather simple distinction was widely adopted both within cuneiform studies and in neighbouring fields, as it conformed to the *Zeitgeist*, which still held an unshakeable belief in the possibility of distinguishing between magic and science in ancient healing practices. However, with the paradigmatic shifts in the cultural sciences, there was also a growing uneasiness with that division in medical cuneiform studies, and in time this led to revision of Ritter's thesis. When Marten Stol addressed the problem in 1992 he showed that studies of Mesopotamian healing must take into account not only the *asû* and the *āšipu*, but also the *bārû* "diviner", and he stressed the use of popular magic by the *asû*.[2] Three years

* I am indebted to Prof. Gernot Wilhelm (Würzburg) for his advice on the date of the letter KBo I 10+, to Prof. John A. Brinkman (Chicago) for information on Rabâ-ša-Marduk, and to Dr. Martin Worthington (Cambridge) for numerous remarks as well as for correcting my English. Any remaining mistakes are, of course, entirely mine.

[1] E. Ritter, "Magical-Expert (=*ĀŠIPU*) and Physician (=*ASÛ*). Notes on Two Complementary Professions in Babylonian Medicine," in *Studies in Honor of Benno Landsberger on his Seventy-Fifth Birthday, April 21, 1965*, eds. H.G. Güterbock and T. Jacobsen, Assyriological Studies 16 (Chicago Oriental Institute: University of Chicago, 1965), 299–321.

[2] M. Stol, "Diagnosis and Therapy in Babylonian Medicine," *Jaarbericht Ex Oriente Lux* 32 (1991–1992): 42–65, esp. 58–62.

later Robert Biggs directly rejected the distinction in terms of the exorcist practicing magic and the physician being rational, stating that "the distinction is more theoretical than real".[3] Recently, JoAnn Scurlock dissented from the distinction into opposites with the following words: "If we cannot separate *asû* and *āšipu*, it is because we are looking for binary opposites where there are not any".[4]

The problem of the distinction between the two Mesopotamian healing professions is an epistemological one: any deductive theory can only be as convincing as its premisses are valid, which means that all theoretical distinctions we make between the *asû* and *āšipu* rest on the quantity and quality of the available sources. Therein lies the core of the problem, for our material is still too scanty to solve this riddle beyond doubt. Apart from the fact that our sources highlight only certain periods, especially the Old Babylonian and Neo-Assyrian epochs, one of the main parts of the enigma is the insufficient connection between the evidence of documents of daily life like letters and receipts on the one hand and the hundreds of extant medical texts on the other.[5] In letters and receipts we see both the *asû* and the *āšipu* as very active healers, sometimes working together, sometimes alone.[6] According to the colophons, however, the medical texts belong almost exclusively to *āšipūtu* "the art of the exorcist".[7] This lack of *asûtu*, the "art of the physician" severely distorts our evidence. However, the paucity of sources for *asûtu* can be attributed to the accident of discovery: whereas two big private libraries belong-

---

[3] R.D. Biggs, "Medicine, Surgery, and Public Health in Ancient Mesopotamia," in *Civilizations of the ancient Near East*, eds. J.M. Sasson et al. (New York: Charles Scribner' Sons, 1995), 1911–1924, esp. 1918.

[4] JA. Scurlock, "Physician, Exorcist, Conjurer, Magician: A Tale of Two Healing Professionals," in *Mesopotamian Magic: Textual, Historical, and Interpretative Perspectives*, eds. T. Abusch and K. van der Toorn, Ancient Magic and Divination 1 (Groningen: Styx Publications 1999), 69–79, esp. 76.

[5] This problem is also addressed in M. Worthington's contribution elsewhere in this volume.

[6] Compare for the Old Babylonian period J.-M. Durand, "Sixième partie : Maladies et médecins", in *Archives Épistolaires de Mari I/1*, ed. J.-M. Durand, Archives Royales de Mari 26/1, 543–584 (Paris: Editions Recherche sur les Civilisations 1988), 541–548 and the sources cited there, and for the Neo-Assyrian period P. Villard, "Les guérisseurs à la cour néo-assyrienne", in *Médecine et médecins au Proche-Orient ancien, Actes du Colloque International organisé à Lyon les 8 et 9 novembre 2002, Maison de l'Orient et de la Méditerranée*, eds. L. Battini et P. Villard (Oxford: John and Erika Hedge Ltd, 2006), 139–160.

[7] H. Hunger, *Babylonische und assyrische Kolophone*, Alter Orient und Altes Testament 2 (Neukirchen-Vluyn: Verlag Butzon & Bercker Kevelaer, 1968), 159 lists only very few tablets that were written by physicians (*asû*) and most of these are not medical.

ing to exorcists were discovered in Assur and in Uruk, no private library belonging to a physician has yet been excavated. As long as we do not find such a physician's library or the library of a temple of Gula, the goddess of healing, we must look for *asûtu*, for physicians, in the tablets we have. In order to present such a medical tablet from Babylonia actually written by a physician, a short detour via the Hittite capital Ḫattuša is necessary.

One of the most interesting pages in the history of Ancient Near Eastern medicine tells of the sending of Babylonian physicians and exorcists to the Hittite court at Ḫattuša in the 14th and 13th centuries B.C. In the famous letter KBo I 10+ addressed to his royal Babylonian "brother" Kadašman-Enlil II, the Hittite Great King Ḫattušili III (ca. 1265–1240 B.C.) tells of a Babylonian physician who shortly after arriving in the Hittite capital fell sick and died. In this context, feeling accused by Kadašman-Enlil that the Hittites detain Babylonian scholars in Hattuša instead of returning them in accordance with the wishes of the Babylonian king, he relates the story of a physician and an exorcist who came to Ḫattuša in the time of his predecessor Muwattalli II (ca. 1290–1272 B.C.) and were not allowed to return to Babylonia. The passage reads thus:[8]

> Thus speak [to my brother]: When they received during the reign of my brother Muwattalli an exorcist and a physician (from Babylonia) and detained them, I was the one to argue with him saying, "Why do you detain them? [To detain an exorcist and a physician] is not according to our custom!" And now I am supposed to have detained your physician? Of the former [experts] whom they had received here, the exorcist is perhaps dead, [the physician Rabâ-ša-Marduk however is] alive. The woman he married here is of my own family and he owns a nice house. [But if he had said] 'I want to leave for my native country', he could have gone right away. [And] *I* am supposed to have held back the physician Rabâ-ša-Marduk?

This prime example of the successful integration of foreigners – at least from the viewpoint of the Hittite Great King Ḫattušili III – has often been translated and cited. And yet, no one hitherto has observed that the name of the physician, Rabâ-ša-Marduk, is extremely rare. This name corresponds to a well known Babylonian type of name (meaning: Great are (the deeds) of Marduk), but for "Rabâ-ša" "great are (the deeds) of"

[8] The translation is based on A.L. Oppenheim's translation in *Letters from Mesopotamia* (Chicago/London, 1967), 145, but incorporates the improvements by E. Edel, *Ägyptische Ärzte und ägyptische Medizin am hethitischen Königshof: neue Funde von Keilschriftbriefen Ramses' II. aus Bogazköy* (Opladen: Westdeutscher Verlag, 1976), 112–123 and A. Hagenbuchner, *Die Korrespondenz der Hethiter II*, Texte der Hethiter 16, (Heidelberg: Carl Winter Universitätsverlag, 1989), 293.

to be connected with the divine name Marduk is very rare. Names like Rabâ-ša-Gula or Rabâ-ša-Ninurta are ubiquitously attested, whereas there are only a handful of instances of the name Rabâ-ša-Marduk. Indeed, so rare is this name, that several of the early translators of this letter, like Hans Martin Kümmel[9] and A. Leo Oppenheim,[10] mistook the name for a title and translated the passage as "great/famous physician of Marduk". They did so, of course, because the vertical wedge, which is used as a determinative for personal names, is missing before this name. However, this happens quite a few times in this particular letter and is *per se* no indication that this cannot be a name. Elmar Edel[11] discussed the problem in his thorough treatment of the letter and came to the conclusion that the title "great physician of Marduk" would be most unusual and without parallel, whereas the name "Rabâ-ša-Marduk" would fit the context perfectly. Edel's position can now be substantiated as three newly published documents from Nippur dating to the Middle Babylonian period mention the name of the famous physician. Most interesting is the receipt of dates UM 29-13-587[12] dated to the eleventh year of king Nazi-Maruttaš who reigned from 1302–1277:

obv

1	2 PI ZÚ.LUM.MA SIG$_5$	Twelve *sūtu* (of) high quality dates
2	^{I}GAL-*šá*-^{d}AMAR.UTU A.ZU	the physician Rabâ-ša-Marduk received
3	*a-na* SISKUR-*šu*	for his sacrifice.
4	*im-ḫur*	
r. 5	^{iti}KIN-^{d}INANNA	Month Ulūlu,
6	U$_4$ 19-KÁM	19th day,
7	MU 11-KÁM	11th year of
8	*Na-zi-Mu-ru-ta*[*š*]	Nazi-Maruttaš.

In yet another receipt for dates dated to the 15th year of Nazi-Maruttaš (CBS 10522+)[13] a certain Rabâ-ša-[is mentioned, who again receives the dates for his sacrifice (*ana nīqišu imḫur*). In the light of the similarity with the afore-mentioned document UM 29-13-587, the recipient of the dates

---

[9] H.M. Kümmel, *Ersatzrituale für den hethitischen König*, Studien zu den Bogazköy-Texten 3 (Wiesbaden: Harrassowitz, 1967), 97 f.

[10] A.L. Oppenheim, *Letters from Mesopotamia* (Chicago/London, 1967), 145.

[11] E. Edel, *Ägyptische Ärzte*, 122–123.

[12] Published by L. Sassmannshausen, *Beiträge zur Verwaltung und Gesellschaft Babyloniens in der Kassitenzeit*, Baghdader Forschungen 21, (Mainz: Philipp von Zabern, 2001), 364, no. 289.

[13] L. Sassmannshausen, *Beiträge*, 365, no. 290.

may well be the same Rabâ-ša-Marduk.[14] A third receipt dated to the 17th year of Nazi-Maruttaš (UM 29-13-291)[15] records the allocation of one mina of tallow for a journey to Babylon to a Rabâ-ša-Marduk whose profession is unfortunately not stated.[16]

It is a commonplace in Assyriology to stress the problems of prosopography, especially the identification of a person by the simple identity of the name. In our case, however, not only does the – rather rarely attested[17] – name match, but the stated professions also agree. The physician Rabâ-ša-Marduk mentioned in the first two cases, perhaps also in the third, corresponds in my view to the physician Rabâ-ša-Marduk who worked in Babylonia and went to Ḫattuša during the reign of Muwattalli II. Furthermore, the historical frame fits nicely, as Nazi-Maruttaš, who ruled from 1302–1277 B.C.,[18] was a contemporary of Muwattalli II, who is dated to about 1290–1272 B.C. In the years 11–17 of Nazi-Maruttaš (corresponding to 1291–1285 B.C.) the physician Rabâ-ša-Marduk lived and worked in Babylonia, and sometime after 1285 B.C. he moved to Ḫattuša in order to serve the Hittite king, where he still dwelled in around 1255–1250 B.C., as stated by the letter of Ḫattušili III.

By connecting these different sources we are able to trace the career of a single physician who was certainly one of the foremost specialists of his time, since otherwise he would not have been selected by the Babylonian king to be sent to the Hittite capital. The documents from Nippur tell

---

[14] L. Sassmannshausen, *Beiträge*, 365 restores the name to ᴵGAL-šá-[ᵈAMAR.UTU].

[15] L. Sassmannshausen, *Beiträge*, 396, no. 339.

[16] A person named Rabâ-ša-Marduk is also mentioned in four unpublished documents from Nippur, which were kindly brought to my attention by Prof. John Brinkman (Chicago): In Ni. 127 the physician Rabâ-ša-Marduk receives food rations "*ana ṣamādi*", the text is dated to the 17th year of an unnamed king. In Ni. 6127 the physician Rabâ-ša-Marduk again receives rations, partly for a journey to Babylon, compare UM 29-13-291, mentioned above. The date of this document is unfortunately lost. A certain ᴵGAL-*šá*-ᵈAMAR.UTU [...] is mentioned in the rations list Ni. 732, which is dated to the year 21 of a king, whose name is broken off.

[17] Apart from these seven instances and the one mentioned below, which very probably all belong to the same Rabâ-ša-Marduk, there are only few other attestations of an individual named Rabâ-ša-Marduk. Two come from Nippur and mention a Rabâ-ša-Marduk in unclear context, see M. Hölscher, *Die Personennamen der kassitischen Texte aus Nippur*, IMGULA 1 (Münster: Rhema-Verlag, 1996), 173. Neither is clearly dated, and it is possible that both refer to the physician Rabâ-ša-Marduk. Certainly a different Rabâ-ša-Marduk is mentioned in CT 10/3: Rev. 24, an inscription from the time of Nabû-apla-iddina.

[18] This date is based on the most recent Babylonian chronology as proposed by J. Boese, "Burnaburiaš II., Melišipak und die mittelbabylonische Chronologie," *Ugarit-Forschungen* 14 (1982): 15–26. These dates correspond to the ones given by H. Gasche et

us that he was active in Babylonia for at least six years, presumably more, before he moved to Ḫattuša, where he stayed at least fifteen years. Fifteen years is the minimum time if we take the last regnal year of Muwattalli II (1272 B.C.) and the first regnal year of Kadašman-Enlil II (1258 B.C.) into account. However, as Rabâ-ša-Marduk presumably left Babylonia only a couple of years after 1285 B.C. and the letter mentioning him was probably not written in the first year of the reign of Kadašman-Enlil II, but more likely around the years 1255–1250,[19] one can speculate that he stayed in Ḫattuša around 25–30 years. By the time the letter of Ḫattušili III to Kadašman-Enlil II was written he must have been quite old, probably looking back on a long medical career mostly spent at the Hittite court.

In spite of the assurance of Ḫattušili III that Rabâ-ša-Marduk is not being detained in Ḫattuša against his will, the truth, as Carlo Zaccagnini[20] has pointed out, may well be very different. Once the Babylonian (and, incidentally, also Egyptian) specialists had arrived at the Hittite court, they seldom, if ever, returned to their native lands. Obviously, as in the case of Rabâ-ša-Marduk, they were tempted into staying abroad by wealth, real-estate properties and even kinship ties with the king, and/or they were simply denied the means to return. This more or less forced stay of scholars at a potentate's court has many parallels in later history,

al., *Dating the Fall of Babylon: A Reappraisal of Second-Millennium Chronology (a joint Ghent-Chicago-Harvard project)*, Mesopotamian History and Environment, Series II, Memoirs, Vol. 4 (Ghent/Chicago: Oriental Institute of the University of Chicago, 1998), timechart, where the article by Boese is not cited.

[19] The date of the letter KBo I 10+ has been a matter of controversy. The decisive point is whether or not the passage obv. 71–75 can be understood as Kadašman-Enlil having diplomatic relations to Egypt in spite of Ḫattušili and Ramses still being at odds. This is the opinion of E. Edel, "Die Abfassungszeit des Briefes KBo I 10 (Ḫattušil – Kadašman-Ellil) und seine Bedeutung für die Chronologie Ramses' II," *Journal of Cuneiform Studies* 12 (1958): 130–133, followed by H. Klengel, *Geschichte des hethitischen Reiches*, Handbuch der Orientalistik, Erste Abteilung, Nahe und der Mittlere Osten 34 (Leiden/Boston, Köln: Brill, 1999), 272. However, as M. Rowton, "The Material From Western Asia and the Chronology of the Nineteenth Dynasty," *Journal of Near Eastern Studies* 25 (1966): 240–258, esp. 243–249, has pointed out, this has the disadvantage that the Hittite-Babylonian alliance in the time of Kadašman-Turgu, the regency of Itti-Marduk-balāṭu and the beginning of Kadašman-Enlil's independent reign are cramped into less than about 6 years. While this is not completely impossible, it is highly unlikely, and therefore we assume that the letter was written some time later, between 1255–1250 B.C. See also A. Hagenbuchner, *Die Korrespondenz der Hethiter II*, Texte der Hethiter 16 (Heidelberg: Carl Winter Universitätsverlag,1989), 295.

[20] C. Zaccagnini, "Patterns of Mobility Among Ancient Near Eastern Craftsmen," *Journal of Near Eastern Studies* 42 (1983): 245–264, esp. 253 f.

which serve to show that this is no isolated case. This is exemplified by the well-known passage in Herodotus telling of the healing of king Darius' injured leg by the famous Greek physician Democedes of Croton, who got a great house and ate at the king's table, but was not allowed to return home.[21] The words of Ḫattušili III, suggesting Rabâ-ša-Marduk might leave whenever he wished to, need not be mendacious, however. Very probably the Hittite king knew perfectly well that the – by now probably more than sixty years old – Babylonian physician had adapted to his new home, where he had family and reputation, and did not plan to leave.

Even if we can trace the career of a distinguished Middle Babylonian physician by combining these different documents, our knowledge is still limited as long as we cannot connect this individual physician to the medical texts that form the basis of our knowledge of Mesopotamian medicine. This might not prove easy, as only a handful of Middle Babylonian medical tablets are extant. However, it is a happy circumstance that among the Middle Babylonian tablets found in the Assyrian capital Assur there is indeed one that can be linked to the physician Rabâ-ša-Marduk. This tablet belongs to those that were brought from Babylonia to Assyria in an attempt to make Assur a centre of learning, providing essential knowledge for the rule of the Assyrian king. Some of these tablets were probably acquired by peaceful means, but the majority were simply looted when Assyrian troops led by the king Tukultī-Ninurta I invaded the north of Babylonia in ca. 1207 B.C. This looting of literary and scientific cuneiform tablets was celebrated as a great success in the famous epic of Tukultī-Ninurta, which was probably commissioned by the king himself.[22] The medical tablet with a connection to Rabâ-ša-Marduk has been known for some time, as Erich Ebeling published it as early as 1920 and Franz Köcher republished it as number 11 in the first volume of his "Babylonisch-assyrische Medizin" in 1963.[23] It is a small

[21] Herodotus III 125–137. Also cited by C. Zaccagnini, *JNES* 42 (1983): 255. See there for additional historical examples.

[22] P. Machinist, "The Epic of Tukulti-Ninurta I: A Study in Middle Assyrian Literature" (unp. PhD Yale University, 1978), 128, lines 2′-11′.

[23] E. Ebeling, *Keilschrifttexte aus Assur religiösen Inhalts*, 2. Band, 1. Heft, Wissenschaftliche Veröffentlichungen der Deutschen Orient-Gesellschaft 34 (Leipzig: J.C. Hinrichs'sche Buchhandlung, 1915–1923), no. 188. F. Köcher, *Die babylonisch-assyrische Medizin in Texten und Untersuchungen* 1 (Berlin: Walter de Gruyter & Co, 1963), no. 11. Apart from these copies, the text was translated by R. Campbell Thompson, *AJSL* 54 (19) 12–16. Parts of it have been transliterated and translated as parallels to other texts by A. Attia and G. Buisson, "Edition de texte: 'Si le crâne d'un homme contient de la chaleur, deuxième tablette'", *Le Journal des Médecines Cunéiformes* 1 (2003): 3–24

broad tablet in fine Middle Babylonian script containing 35 lines and a three-line colophon. The colophon summarizes the tablet's 18 prescriptions as follows:

36 Eighteen prescriptions for headache (lit.: seizing of the temple).
37 First Tablet
38 From the hand of Rabiā-ša-Marduk

Here, the uncontracted form Rabiā instead of the contracted form Rabâ is used (GAG § 113 d), but the same name is meant. The profession of the writer Rabiā/Rabâ-ša-Marduk is not stated, but it is highly likely that he was a healer. The hypothesis suggests itself that it was precisely our Rabâ-ša-Marduk who wrote this tablet during his time in Babylonia at the turn from the 14th to 13th century, and that it stayed behind when he left for Ḫattuša. Almost a century later, when Tukultī-Ninurta invaded Babylonia, it was brought to Assur together with other scientific tablets.

Documents Mentioning the Physician Rabâ-ša-Marduk

Babylonia		**Ḫattuša**
In the years 11–17 (1291–1285) of Nazi-Maruttaš (1302–1277) several receipts from Nippur mention Rabâ-ša-Marduk in Babylonia	↘	
		After 1285, during the reign of Muwattalli II (ca. 1290–1272), Rabâ-ša-Marduk moves to Ḫattuša (Kbo I 10+)
		↓
		Around 1255–1250 Ḫattušili III writes to Kadašman-Enlil and mentions Rabâ-ša-Marduk (KBo I 10+)
	↙	
Around 1207 Tukultī-Ninurta I loots the medical tablet of Rabâ-ša-Marduk (BAM 11) and transfers it to Assur		

---

and by JA. Scurlock, *Magico-Medical Means of Treating Ghost-Induced Illnesses in Ancient Mesopotamia*, Ancient Magic and Divination 3 (Leiden/Boston: Brill-Styx, 2006), 700 f. As there has never been a transliteration and translation of the whole tablet, it is edited here in the appendix.

If the Rabiā-ša-Marduk of BAM 11 is indeed identical with the Rabâ-ša-Marduk of the aforementioned documents, and the present writer has little doubt about it, then we have a date for the undated tablet, which must have been written shortly after the year 1300 B.C., some time between 1300 and 1280. This is revealing in so far as the tablet shows a distinct logographic style and its syllabary points to the syllabic conventions of the first millennium B.C.[24] But what is more, we can now show that the tablet BAM 11 was with all probability not written by an exorcist but by a physician. At first glance this seems to be a marginal point, but a closer look at the text is interesting.

Several of the prescriptions on BAM 11 have parallels in the later therapeutic series *šumma amēlu muḫḫašu umma ukāl*, which we know mainly from the seventh century libraries of Ashurbanipal in Niniveh. Ten of the eighteen prescriptions duplicate the second tablet of the series *šumma amēlu muḫḫašu umma ukāl*, often simply called UGU 2. Annie Attia and Gilles Buisson naturally included BAM 11 in their recent edition of the second tablet of UGU as manuscript D,[25] yet one should not be mistaken in that this Middle Babylonian text is not part of the series but rather contains some of the same prescriptions.

BAM 11 vs. UGU 2

BAM 11	UGU 2
(obv.) 1–3	1–4
—	< 1 prescription
4–6	7–9
7–8	10–12
9	13–14
—	< 1 prescription
10–11	17–18

[24] For the logographic style compare the edition in the appendix (passim), and for the syllabic conventions note the use of the sign ŠÚ (rev. 30) for the 3rd person pronominal suffix which is not often so used in Middle Babylonian texts. The phonetic value *tara* of the sign TAR in verbal forms like *tara-bak* (obv. 2) and *tara-kás* (obv. 17, rev. 33) is not noted for Middle Babylonian texts in W. von Soden and W. Röllig, *Das akkadische Syllabar, 4th ed.*, Analecta Orientalia 42, (Roma, Pontificio Istituto Biblico: 1991), 3, just as the phonetic value *kás* of the sign BI is not (Syllabar, p. 26).

[25] A. Attia and G. Buisson, *JMC* 1 (2003): 3–24.

<table>
<tr><th>BAM 11</th><th>UGU 2</th></tr>
<tr><td>12–13</td><td>19–20</td></tr>
<tr><td>14–15</td><td>21–22</td></tr>
<tr><td>16–17</td><td>—</td></tr>
<tr><td>18</td><td>—</td></tr>
<tr><td>(rev.) 19–20</td><td>66–67</td></tr>
<tr><td>21–22</td><td rowspan="5">DIŠ LÚ GIDIM DAB-su-ma
SAG.KI.DAB.BA TUK.TUK</td></tr>
<tr><td>23–24</td></tr>
<tr><td>25–26</td></tr>
<tr><td>27</td></tr>
<tr><td>28–29</td></tr>
<tr><td>30–31</td><td>—</td></tr>
<tr><td>32–33</td><td>49–50</td></tr>
<tr><td>—</td><td>< 2 prescriptions</td></tr>
<tr><td>34–35</td><td>54–55</td></tr>
</table>

A short look at the parallels between the eighteen prescriptions and UGU 2 shows that the first fifteen lines of BAM 11 duplicate the beginning of UGU 2, though UGU 2 inserts two more prescriptions after the first and fourth prescription on BAM 11. There are three more parallels to UGU 2 on the reverse of BAM 11, but eight prescriptions on BAM 11 are not to be found in the preserved portions of UGU 2.[26] The five prescriptions of lines 21–29 begin differently, mentioning the seizure by a ghost, and might well have been incorporated into one of the ghost-tablets, although no duplicates to these prescriptions can be found.[27] However, it is astonishing that, for example, the prescription of lines 30–31, starting with the symptoms *šumma amīlu tīb pūti* (or *nakkapti*) *iraššši u zumuršu ikkalšu* "If a man gets a pulsating temple and his body hurts him", was not incorporated into UGU 2, although one would expect it there. This text represents, therefore, the kind of "forerunner", which an editor of a new series would incorporate into his new series, selecting the prescriptions

[26] Admittedly, around 35 lines of UGU 2 are still lost: see A. Attia and G. Buisson, *JMC* 1 (2003): 7, after l. 108 and 8, after l. 138′. However, it is unlikely that all the prescriptions on BAM 11 which are missing from UGU 2 are to be restored in these lacunae.

[27] JA. Scurlock, *Magico-Medical Means of Treating Ghost-Induced Illnesses in Ancient Mesopotamia*, Ancient Magic and Divination 3 (Leiden/Boston: Brill-Styx, 2006), nos. 55–56, and nos. 62–64.

according to his own understanding of relevance and sequence, adopting one passage while rejecting another. However, the fact that so many of the prescriptions of BAM 11, a text which was very probably copied, if not composed, by a physician, were incorporated into the big medical therapeutic series that was copied and worked on by exorcists, shows that both professions could draw upon the same texts.

One could note here that the eighteen prescriptions of BAM 11 do not include any incantations, but this would not do justice to the problem as UGU 2 does not contain any incantations either. Furthermore, some ingredients in the prescriptions on BAM 11 are what we consider 'magical' components, like the risp of date-palm that rustles, or old grease from the city gate. It is not so much the presence or absence of magic that makes BAM 11 so interesting, but the fact that it was written by a physician and that – according to the colophon – it was the first tablet of an unnamed series. This is more than just a hint for the existence of an older therapeutic series, which was already similar to the later UGU-series. Like other textual genres, such as divinatory texts or the lexical lists, some medical therapeutic medical texts seem to have been formed into series in Middle Babylonian times. Furthermore, it is not impossible that the tablet BAM 11 records an original composition by Rabâ-ša-Marduk, and not one copied from another tablet, for the colophon does not state any copying and nothing within the text, like a *ḫi-pí* "broken"-remark, supports the idea of a copy. If this is indeed an original, then the physician Rabâ-ša-Marduk would be one of the famous medical practitioners whose knowledge and experience laid the foundation for the late medical therapeutic series *šumma amēlu muḫḫašu umma ukāl*, which can be regarded as the legacy of cuneiform medicine.

Appendix: Edition of VAT 10267 (KAR 188, BAM 11)

VAT 10267 is the major part of a horizontally oriented tablet measuring 64 × 104 mm. The lower right edge is broken away, but the tablet is otherwise well preserved. It is written in a fine Middle Babylonian ductus. The 18 prescriptions are separated by single rulings which tend to slope upwards at each end of the line. The colophon appears on the upper edge without being highlighted by rulings, but is indented by about 2.5 cm.

Transliteration:

Obv.

1 DIŠ LÚ SAG.KI.DAB.BA TUK.TUK NUMUN ÚKUŠ.LAGAB NUMUN ÚKUŠ.TI.GI.⌜IL⌝ NUMUN ^{ú}EME.UR.GI$_7$ NUMUN ^{ú}*e-di*

2 NUMUN ^{giš}KIRI$_6$ NUMUN *kiš-ša-ni* TÉŠ.BI GAZ SIM *ma-al-ma-liš* ḪE.ḪE *i+na* A.GEŠTIN.NA *tara-bak*

3 ZÌ ŠE.SA.A ZÌ ZÍZ.AN.NA *a-na pa-ni ta-ša-ba-aḫ i+na* KUŠ *te-ṭer-ri* SAG.DU-*su tu-gal-lab* LAL-*ma* TI.LA

---

4 DIŠ KI.MIN ^{giš}EREN ^{giš}ŠUR.MÌN ^{giš}ŠIM.GÍR! GI.DÙG.GA ^{šim}LI ^{šim}KU$_7$.KU$_7$ ^{šim}*šu-pu-uḫ-*[*ru*]

5 ^{šim}MUG ŠIM.SAL ^{šim}IM.DU ^{šim}ḪAB ILLU *ba-lu-ḫi* TÉŠ.BI GAZ [SIM]

6 *i+na* GEŠTIN SUR.RA *ta-rab-bak* ZÌ ŠE.SA.A ZÌ ZÍZ.AN.NA *a-na* IGI *ta-ša-ba-aḫ* x [ ]

---

7 DIŠ KI.MIN NUMUN ^{giš}ÍLDAG ^{ú}*ak-tam* NUMUN ÁB.DUḪ ^{ú}*am-ḫa-ra* GAZI^{sar} NUMUN ^{giš}Ḫ[AB]

8 *i+na* GEŠTIN SUR.RA *ta-rab-ba-ak* [LAL-*ma* TI.LA]

---

9 DIŠ KI.MIN ^{ú}ḪAR.ḪAR ^{ú}KUR.KUR ^{ú}*ak-tam* NUMUN ÁB.DUḪ ZÌ GIG DIDA S[IG$_5$]

---

10 DIŠ KI.MIN ^{šim}KU$_7$.KU$_7$ ^{šim}LI ŠIM ^{d}*Nin-urta* ZÌ GIG [ ]

11 *i+na* KAŠ.SAG *ta-la-aš tu-ba-a'-a-rù* SAG.D[U-*su tu-gal-lab* LAL-*ma* TI.LA]

---

12 DIŠ KI.MIN ^{šim}KU$_7$.KU$_7$ ^{šim}LI ŠIM ^{d}*Nin-urta* N[UMUN ÁB.DUḪ KA A.AB.BA]

13 ^{šim}MUG TÉŠ.BI GAZ SIM *i+na* KA[Š *ta-rab-bak*]

---

14 DIŠ KI.MIN ^{giš}PA GIŠIMMAR *ša i+na-zu-zu* ŠU.TI *t*[*u-*]

15 *i+na* A GAZI^{sar} *ta-la-aš* L[AL-*ma* TI.LA]

---

16 DIŠ LÚ ZI-*ib* SAG.KI TUK ^{giš}PA GIŠIM[MAR]

17 *i+na* ^{sík}ḪÉ.ME.DA *tara-kás* [ ]

---

18 DIŠ KI.MIN SA MAŠ.DÀ ^{sík}ḪÉ.ME.DA MUNUS x [ ]

---

lower edge

Rev.

19 *ana* ZI-*ib* SA SAG.KI *nu-uḫ-ḫi* DUḪ.ŠE.[GIŠ.Ì]
20 *i+na* ZÌ.KUM DIDA *ù* KAŠ.SA[G ŠEG$_6$.GA *tara-bak* LAL-*ma* TI.LA]

---

21 DIŠ LÚ GIDIM DAB-*su-ma* SAG.KI.DAB.BA TUK.TUK x [ ]
22 *tu-ba-aḫ-ḫa-ar ba-aḫ-ru-su* [ ]

---

23 DIŠ LÚ GIDIM DAB-*su-ma* SAG.KI.DAB.BA TUK.TUK ^{giš}GEŠ[TIN.KA$_5$.A$^?$]
24 *i+na* A GAZI^{sar} *ta-la-aš* [LAL-*ma* TI.LA]

---

25 DIŠ KI.MIN Ì.SUMUN *ša* ^{giš}IG KÁ.GAL *i+na* È-*ka a-na* ZAG-*k*[*a* GUB-*zu* TI-*qé*]
26 GE$_6$ U$_4$ BI DUR NU.NU *i+na* ^{sík}ÀKA NIGIN-*m*[*a ina* SAG.KI-*šú* KEŠDA]

---

27 DIŠ KI.MIN SUḪUŠ ^{giš}DÌḪ NIGIN-*ma ta-na-saḫ* ^{sík}ḪÉ.ME.DA NU.NU [ ]

---

28 DIŠ KI.MIN LAG.A.ŠÀ.GA ^{giš}ZA.BA.LAM ZÌ ŠE.SA.A DUḪ.ŠE.GIŠ.Ì [ ]
29 ^{šim}LI TÉŠ.BI GAZ SIM 1/3 SÌLA-TA.ÀM *i+na* KAŠ.SAG x [ ]

---

30 DIŠ LÚ ZI-*ib* SAG.KI TUK *ù* SU$^!$(text: zu)-*šú* GU$_7$-*šú* ^{giš}PA MES.MÁ.KAN.NA ḪÁD.DU G[AZ SIM ZÌ GÚ.GAL]
31 ZÌ GÚ.TUR ZÌ ŠE.IN.NU.ḪA *i+na šur-šum-mi* KAŠ.SAG LAL.LAL-*su-ma* T[I.LA]

---

32 DIŠ LÚ ZI-*ib* SAG.KI TUK *ù ri-mu-ta$_5$* TUK PA ^{giš}ḪÉNBUR.A ḪÁD.DU GAZ SIM Z[Ì ŠE.MUŠ$_5$]
33 *saḫ-lé-e ṭe$_4$-ne-e-ti* ZÌ ŠE.SA.A TÉŠ.BI ḪE.ḪE *i+na* A GAZI^{sar} *tara-bak* LAL.L[AL-*ma* TI.LA]

---

34 DIŠ LÚ ZI-*ib* SAG.KI TUK *ù šim-ma-ta$_5$* TUK ^{giš}PA MA.NU ḪÁD *ta-sàk* ZÌ G[IG]
35 *saḫ-lé-e* ^{ú}ḪAR.ḪAR *i+na* KAŠ LÚ.KURUN.NA *ta-rab-bak* LAL.LAL-*su-ma* TI.LA

Colophon:

36 18 *bu-ul-ṭú ša* SAG.KI.DAB.BA
37 IM.GÍD.DA 1-KAM.MA
38 *ša* ŠU$^!$ *Ra-bi-a-ša-^{d}*AMAR.UTU

Translation:

1–3 If a man regularly gets headache (literally: seizing of the temple), you crush together seeds of *errû*, seeds of *tigilû*, seeds of *cynoglossum*, seeds of *ēdu*-plant, seeds of the garden, (and) seeds of *kiššānu*-peas, you sieve it, you mix it in equal parts, you mix it with vinegar into a paste, powdered roasted barley (and) emmer flour you sprinkle on it, rub it onto a skin, shave his head, bind it on and he will recover.

4–6 If ditto, you crush together cedar-wood, cypress-wood, myrtle, 'sweet-reed', juniper, *kukru*-aromatic, cedar-resin, *ballukku*-aromatic, *šimšalû*-aromatic, *suādu*-aromatic, opoponax (and) resin of *baluḫḫu*-plant, [you sieve it], you mix it with must into a paste, powdered roasted barley (and) emmer flour you sprinkle on it, … […].

7–8 If ditto, [you crush together] seed of *ildakku*-wood, *aktam*-plant, *kammantu*-seed, *amḫara*-plant, *kasû*, seed of *ḫu*[*rātu* … …], you mix it with must into a paste, [bind it on and he will recover].

9 If ditto, [… …] *ḫašû*-plant, *atā'išu*-plant, *aktam*-plant, *kammantu*-seed, wheat flour, good quality *billatu*-beer [… …].

10–11 If ditto, you knead *kukru*-aromatic, juniper, Ninurta-aromatic, wheat flour [… …] in beer, you heat (it), [shave his] head, [bind it on and he will recover].

12–13 If ditto, you crush together *kukru*-aromatic, juniper, Ninurta-aromatic, s[eed of *kammantu*, *imbū tâmtim*-mineral], *ballukku*-aromatic, you sieve it, you mix it with bee[r into a paste … …].

14–15 If ditto, you take the risp of date-palm that rustles, you [… …] you knead it with extract of *kasû*, you b[ind it on and he will recover].

16–17 If a man gets a pulsating of the temple, the risp of a date-[palm … …], you bind it with red wool [… …].

18 If ditto, the sinew of a gazelle, red wool, … [… …].

19–20 In order to ease a pulsating of the vein of the temple, [you mix] sesa[me left overs … …] with *isqūqu*-flour, *billatu*-beer and [boiled?] bee[r into a paste, bind it on and he will recover].

21–22 If a ghost seizes a man so that he continually has a headache, you heat [… …], still hot [… …].

23–24 If a ghost seizes a man so that he continually has a headache, you knead [fox] gr[ape? ...] with extract of *kasû*, [you bind it on and he will recover].

25–26 If ditto, [you take] old grease from the door of the city gate, [(the one which) stands] on your right when you are going out [...] (that) night (and) that day, you twine (it) together into a cord. You wrap (the grease) in a tuft of wool an[d bind it on his temple].

27 If ditto, you cover and uproot root of camel-thorn, you twine (it) together with red-dyed wool [... ...].

28–29 If ditto, you crush together "field clod"-plant, *supālu*-wood, powdered roasted barley, residue of sesame, [...] (and) juniper, you sieve it, a third of *qû*-measure each in beer ... [... ...].

30–31 If a man gets a pulsating of the temple and his body hurts him, you cr[ush and sieve] dried *musukannu*-tree leaves, [*ḫallūru*-pea flour], *kakku*-pea flour (and) *inninu*-barley flour in beer dregs, you bandage him continually (with them) and he will re[cover].

32–33 If a man gets a pulsating of the temple and also *rimūtu*-paralysis, you crush and sieve dried *supālu*-tree leaves, with [*šigūšu*-flo]ur, ground *saḫlû* (and) roasted grain flour you mix it together, with extract of *kasû* you mix it into a paste, you bind (him) con[tinually (with it) and he will recover].

34–35 If a man gets a pulsating of the temple and has numbness, you grind dried *e'ru*-tree leaves, mix it with wh[eat] flour, *saḫlû* (and) *ḫašû*-plant (and) with beer of a tavern keeper into a paste, you bandage him continually (with them) and he will recover].

Colophon:

36 Eighteen prescriptions for headache (lit.: seizing of the temple)
37 First Tablet
38 From the hand of Rabiā-ša-Marduk

Commentary:

4 On collation, the sign copied by Köcher as TAR looks rather different from TAR, but is not a clear GÍR either.

5 For IM.DU as a logographic writing of the plant *suādu* see CAD S 338ff., but cf. AHw 211a for a possible syllabic reading as *em-du*.

10 "Ninurta-aromatic" is often used as a name for the *nikiptu*-plant.

11 The verbal form *tu-ba-a'-a-rù* is very odd, as one expects *tu-ba-aḫ-ḫa-ar* as in l. 22, cf. already AHw 96a and CAD B 307a. The

duplicate AMT 20/1 iv 6′ has *tu-ba-har*, which strongly suggests that *tu-ba-a'-a-rù* derives from *buḫḫuru*. However, the final vowel *u* is hard to explain, and one is tempted to assume a scribal mistake, e.g. in form of a slip as the preceding verbal form ends with the sign AŠ.

18 A possible restoration MUNUS.AN[ŠE …] at the end of the line has been rejected due to semantic difficulties.

25 For the restoration of this line see JA. Scurlock, AMD III, 264.

27 For the practice of covering of plants before uprooting them, so that the plant cannot "see" who is uprooting it, see E. Reiner, *Astral Magic in Babylonia* (Philadelphia: The American Philosophical Society, 1995), 36–38.

31 Collation shows that the last sign is clearly T[I, contrary to the copy of Köcher, BAM 11.

32+34 The pleonastic repetition of TUK might be due to the set phrase ZI-*ib* SAG.KI TUK which also appears in the preceding prescription, in line 30.

38 The second sign in this line is not a perfect ŠU, but looks like the sign SI. However, with H. Hunger, *BAK* p. 34, no. 66 it is considered here to be a variant to the sign ŠU.

"TO BE ILL" IN AKKADIAN: THE VERB *SALĀ'U* AND THE SUBSTANTIVE *SILI'TU*

Marten Stol

There are two words for "to be ill" in Akkadian: *marāṣu* and *salā'u*. The substantives derived from these verbs, globally meaning "disease", are *murṣu* and *sili'tu* (and occasionally *masla'tu*). The first pair, *marāṣu* and *murṣu*, is widely attested, and the verb has cognates in other Semitic languages, where it also means "to be ill" (for example in epigraphic South Arabic). In this contribution, I will concentrate on the second pair.

The verb *salā'u* has been translated in various ways, but nobody has discussed it.[1] W. von Soden's German dictionary (*AHw*) translates "(be)-sprengen, infizieren, überschütten" and remarks that the word may be a "differentiation" of *salāḫu* I, "(Wasser) sprengen". Not written in von Soden's telegraphic style and offering full translations of the meaningful passages, the Chicago Assyrian Dictionary (*CAD*) gives more room for interpretation and reflection. Like the others, the new dictionary *CDA* distinguishes *salāḫu* "to sprinkle" from *salā'u*, which it translates "to sprinkle, slander".

We suggest that *salā'u* and *salāḫu* should not be distinguished, i.e. that there is only one verb, *salā'u*, which has the basic meaning "to sprinkle" and several more specialised meanings derived from the notion of sprinkling. The reason why the phantom verb *salāḫu* was thought to exist is that in the Old Babylonian period the cuneiform script did not yet have signs indicating the combinations vowel+ʾalef or ʾalef+vowel, such as arise in forms of *salā'u*. Instead, the ʾalef was expressed either by using the letter *ḫ*, or by creating a hiatus.[2] Thus in Old Babylonian

[1] N. Heeßel, *Babylonisch-assyrische Diagnostik*, Alter Orient und Altes Testament 43 (Münster: Ugarit Verlag, 2000), 191 note 41, "unklar". M.J. Geller, "An Akkadian Vademecum in the Babylonian Talmud," in *From Athens to Jerusalem, Medicine in Hellenized Jewish Lore and in Early Christian Literature*, eds. S. Kottek and M. Horstmanshoff (Rotterdam: Erasmus Publishing, 2000), 18 note 22, saw a link with Aramaic *ṣilḥ^{a}tā*, "migraine".

[2] Another example of a verb with ʾalef as the final radical is *mašā'u* "to rob, plunder"; this is also spelled with *ḫ* in Old Babylonian.

the forms of the verb *salā'u* are written as if they were forms of a verb *salāḫu*, and the same applies to derived forms: the substantive *sili'tu* is written *siliḫtu*. In later periods, forms and derivatives of *salā'u* can be written with signs in the 'aleph range, but owing to orthographic conservatism they are sometimes still written with signs in the *ḫ* range, and indeed one finds variants with 'aleph and *ḫ* in manuscripts of the same composition (e.g. Ištar's Descent 118 *is-luḫ-ši-ma* var. *is-lu-u'-ši-ma*)

salā'u *in Old Babylonian and Old Assyrian*

In the Old Babylonian period the verb *salā'u* (written as if it were *salāḫu*) is attested with the literal meaning "to sprinkle" in the following contexts:

- "To sprinkle" is used for a kind of irrigation, as Mari scholars pointed out; "faire l'arrosage".[3]
- It is said of barley: "In the whole house the barley is "sprinkled" (= damp?) ([š]e-*um su-lu-uḫ*), there is nothing" (OBTIV 15: 11–13). Barley as fodder and rations, is characterised "from the barley for sprinkling" (šà *še-im ša sà-la-i-im*) (OBTIV 149: 8; month XI; Kiskissum).

The verb *salā'u* also has a metaphoric meaning based on "to sprinkle", i.e. to sprinkle with evil. In Old Assyrian letters this means: "with evil words": "(mit Vorwürfen) überschütten" (*AHw*).[4] Other English translations, such as "to bespatter", "to criticize", look like acceptable translations, but "to slander" (*CDA*) is too strong.

---

[3] AbB 10 177: 26 (*islu'*), 38 (*ina sili'tim la* [...]), in a context of irrigating (*makārum*) and canal digging; D. Charpin, "Compte rendu du CAD volume S (1984)," *Archiv für Orientforschung* 40–41 (1993–1994): 7a. Note in the same letter AbB 10 177: 11 *mi-im-ma* ZA-LA-AŠ+DIŠ-AD (= *sala'at* = ?) *ul ibašši*. In Mari texts J.-M. Durand, *Archives Épistolaires de Mari I/1*, Archives Royales de Mari 26/1 (Paris: Editions Recherche sur les Civilisations 1988), 339 note 20: "*salāḫum* semble être limité à l'usage d'"asperger' en babylonien, alors que dans la langue de Mari, il doit désigner une certaine sorte d'irrigation." Note *mê sullu'* in ARM 3 79 rev. 8, with J.-M. Durand, *Les Documents épistolaires du palais de Mari*, Littératures anciennes du Proche-Orient 17/II, (Paris: Éditions du Cerf, 1998), 596 note g.

[4] AHw 1015a *salā'u* I G 3. Cf. E. Bilgiç and C. Günbattı, *Ankaraner Kültepe-Texte III: Texte der Grabungskampagne 1970*, Freiburger Altorientalische Studien, Beiheft 3 (Stuttgart: Franz Steiner Verlag, 1995), 96 no. 62: 28, 42, with comments.

Four Old Babylonian letters have the warning *la tasalla' / la isalla'*. *AHw* and *CAD* interpret this form as the passive N-stem (*tassalla', issalla'*), but the letter *s* is never written double.

(1) "As to Ibbija: Does the garden have ...? Establish the truth (*bīr*). Do not be critical" (UET 5 12: 19–22) (Ur).

(2) In another letter: *ana bābtija la isalla'*, "he should not be critical about my outstanding payment (?)" (AbB 8 77: 15f.). Or (with the reading of *CAD* S 97a): *ana zum*[*r*]*ija la isalla'*, "he should not be critical towards me (lit. my body)". W. von Soden, in his review of AbB 8, remarks: "*salāḫum* "(Wasser) sprengen" ist hier ohne Objekt absolut gebraucht".[5] This negative command indeed never has an object; as in the following examples:

(3) "[Do not] be critical" (UET 5 72 Left Edge I 1);[6]

(4) "Do not be critical" (*la ta-sà-la-a*[*ḫ*]) (AbB 13 1: 19). *AHw* translates these passages basically as "infiziert werden" (moralisch-politisch): "Laß dich nicht infiziert werden!". *CAD* does not translate it.

I believe that the only reference given for the G-stem in *CAD* S 96a, *ṣuḫāru sali'ma* in an Old Babylonian letter (AbB 6 201: 6, 24), means "the boy has been criticized", not "the boy is ill". Nothing in the letter points to illness.

In a letter from Mari, king Samsi-Addu asks his son to send back the three supernumerary cooks that they do not need: "If you do not send me those men, it is to be feared that future (*warkûtum*) cooks will be criticized (*is-sà-al-la-ḫu*)" (ARM 1 14: 19–22). All scholars agree that a "metaphoric" meaning for *salā'u* N must be assumed in this passage and in this they start from the basic meaning "to be sick, "to be infected".[7] This is wrong, since one should start from the meaning "to sprinkle".

---

[5] W. von Soden, "Review of: I. Cagni, *Briefe aus dem Iraq Museum* (TIM II)," *Bibliotheca Orientalis* 39 (1982): 134b, on Nr. 77 Z. 16.

[6] In UET 5 72 Left Edge I 1 one sees clearly, with AHw: [*la*] *ta-sà-la-aḫ*. CAD S 97a emends this into [*a-di*] *a*(!)-*la-kam*. Is this reading based on a collation? Lines 30f. were collated for CAD; see M/2 146b. Note in Left Edge II 1 *la ta-šu-uš* (not in AHw or CAD).

[7] W. von Soden, "Zu den politischen Korrespondenzen des Archivs von Mâri", *Or NS* 21 (1952): 77 ("anstecken, infizieren", hier in übertragener Bedeutung!); J.-M. Durand, *Les Documents épistolaires du palais de Mari*, Littératures anciennes du Proche-Orient 16/I (Paris: Éditions du Cerf, 1997), 95f. ("les prochains cuisiniers ne soient pas contaminés (par l'exemple)"); N. Wasserman, "The particle *assurre/ē* in the Mari Letters", *Recueil d'études à la mémoire de Maurice Birot*, eds. D. Charpin et J.-M. Durand, Florilegium marianum II, Mémoires de N.A.B.U. 3 (Paris: SEPOA, 1994), 329 with note 53 ("the above mentioned cooks might get a bad example").

Another letter offers according to the copy: "Please! I have been under criticism" (*at-ta-as-li-iḫ*) (TIM 1 20: 83).[8]

Another metaphorical meaning of *salā'u* is disease-related: a sick person is "sprinkled" with disease (a parallel is the idea that disease can "rain down" from heaven[9]), so that passive forms of *salā'u* (G stative, N) mean "to be ill".

The verb *salāḫu* clearly refers to illness in two cautionary clauses in labour contracts. The first passage was so interpreted by *CAD*: "if they (the hired workers) die (ba(!).BAD) or get sick (*i-sà-la-ḫu-ú-ma*), he (nonetheless) pays the rent of the field" (UET 5 204: 11) (Ur). The second text is a contract in the archive of Samija (Sippar), transliterated by Els Woestenburg. Illilum hires from Samija his son for one year. "If he will be ill (or) he will stop working (*naparkû*), he (= Samija) shall pay the silver" (BM 97571: 9 [= rev. 1]; *i-sà-la-aḫ i-pa-ra-ku-ú*). Two handbooks with contract formulas indeed mention "to be ill" in this clause, but in other terms: ù tu.ra ba.an.tu, or ù tu.ra ba.ab.ag, Akkadian *u imtarṣu* (after "he has stopped working", *ittaparkâ*).[10] This clause does not refer to a short disease, but to a lasting disease preventing the hired man from performing his work.

This is confirmed by the discovery of a word which Durand read *sāliḫu* and interpreted as a participle meaning "someone who performs the action of being diseased", but for which we prefer the passive form *salīḫu* "a sprinkled (i.e. diseased) person" (as suggested by Martin Worthington); the word has the same structure as *pašīšum* "an anointed person". The word has the meaning "diseased" in Mari, where these persons are part of men unable to go on campaign;[11] elsewhere, four of

---

[8] A. al-Zeebari, "Altbabylonische Briefe des Iraq-Museums," (Dissertation zur Erlangung des Doktorgrades des Philospohischen Fakultät des Westfälischen Wilhelms-Universität zu Münster 1964), 50, 53 no. 20: 83 ("Bitte, ich wurde angesteckt"); K. Reiter, *Die Metalle im Alten Orient: unter besonderer Berücksichtigung altbabylonischer Quellen*, Alter Orient und Altes Testament 249 (Münster: Ugarit Verlag, 1997), 92*, 95*, 103* ("Bitte, enttäusche mich nicht"; *la ta-as-⟨sa⟩-li-iḫ*).

[9] M. Stol, *Epilepsy in Babylonia*, Cuneiform Monographs 2 (Groningen: Styx Publications, 1993), 12–14, "Diseases from heaven".

[10] M.T. Roth, with a contribution by H.A. Hoffner *Law Collections from Mesopotamia and Asia Minor*, Writings from the Ancient World Series 6 (Atlanta: Scholars Press, 1995) (2nd ed. 1997, corr. reprint 2000), 53 SLHF VIII 7 f., and MSL 1 (1937) 103 Ai VII iv 19.

[11] ARM 3 19: 27, with J.-M. Durand, *Les Documents épistolaires du palais de Mari*, Littératures anciennes du Proche-Orient 17/II (Paris: Éditions du Cerf, 1998), 182.

them are unable to work on the fields.[12] J.-M. Durand distinguishes between this *sāli'um* "souffreteux, de condition chétive", and *marṣum* "malade".

"To be ill" (*salā'um*) and "illness" (*sili'tum*) are attested in a number of letters from which we cannot learn much. Two Old Babylonian letters from one archive in Sippar refer to "the illness falling under the expertise of the doctor" (*si-li-iḫ-ti a-sú-ti*). The first passage says that the writer is "ill of it" (*marṣāku*); it affects his kidneys in some way (*ù ka-li-a-ti-ja ka-aq-qá-rum i-ta-ú*).[13] The second passage is more difficult; my provisional translation is: "Even if they diagnose (*li-du-ma*; verb *idû*) *sili'ti asûti* in his body (*zumru*) and confine him within the city gates (ká.gal.ḫi.a *lu šu-du*), he should not die in imprisonment (*mēseru*)".[14]

A later oracle text distinguishes "the illness falling under the expertise of the doctor, the illness [falling under the expertise of the conjuror], a rare disease, a rare illness".[15]

A Disease of Women?

Two disbursements of sheep for extispicy (Sippar) indicate that this is done "when the Princess had fallen ill (*i-nu-ma* dumu.SAL lugal *is-sà-al-ḫu*)". One of them is dated to month VIII, day 24, the other to month IX (day broken off).[16]

More OB references speak of a woman suffering from this kind of disease. Best known is the legal verdict about what happened during the pregnancy of a woman (PBS 5 100 III 5). The line in question has been translated in various ways. "When Sin-nada, the wife of E., saw (that) 'I am pregnant!' (?) (lit. 'My belly!'), because of E. her husband, he/she repeatedly fell ill" (M. Stol). "When Sin-nada, the wife of E., saw the (pregnant) womb (and revealed it) to E., her husband, she was always falling ill" (*CAD* S 97a; E. Leichty). "When Sin-nada, the wife

[12] TH 84.26: 23, D. Charpin, *AfO* 40–41 (1993–1994): 8b, reviewing CAD S 99.

[13] C. Janssen, "*E'iltam paṭārum : awat hadê !*" in *Mésopotamie et Elam. Actes de la XXXVIe R.A.I. Gand 10–14 juillet 1989*, MHE Occasional Publications 1 (Ghent: University of Ghent, 1991), 101 f. Di 450: 8,10, with p. 93.

[14] Janssen, *ibidem*, 104 Di 628: 15 with p. 92 f.

[15] AMT 17,9: 6–7, "restored from K. 2617+"; thus CAD S 264a, see the new edition by W.G. Lambert, *Babylonian Oracle Questions*, Mesopotamian Civilization 13 (Winona Lake, IN: Eisenbrauns, 2007), 40, no. 1: 336 f.

[16] A. Goetze, "Thirty Tablets from the Reigns of Abī-ešuḫ and Ammī-ditānā", *Journal of Cuneiform Studies* 2 (1948): 77, 104, no. 6; CBS 141, transliterated by Els Woestenburg.

of E., realized my concern for her husband, E., she became depressed" (M.T. Roth; cf. *CAD* S 97a, 2). "Als (?) Sin-nada, die Ehefrau des E., 'mein Herz für ihren Ehemann E. sah', wurde er (/ sie?) immer wieder ...", with the suggestion "bekam er immer wieder Krämpfe" (C. Wilcke, referring to *AHw salāḫu* II).[17]

An oracle for a woman in confinement (*tamīt ḫarištu* [sic]) describes her condition, and again we see the verb *salā'u* N: "Every day she is overwhelmed (*ik-kát-ta-mu*), she is ill (*is-sal-la-'u*), bread and beer are displeasing (*šu*[*m-ru-ṣu*]) to her, her appetite has diminished, her disease [...]".[18]

It is possible that this oracle originally is Old Babylonian.

However, in letters, both men and women are affected by this illness: "That Damiqtum [a woman] is ill (*sa-al-ḫ*[*a-at*]), S. told me. (...) Send me a report of her illness, that I should not worry (*nakādu*)" (AbB 10 210: 3–6, 11–13). "He said: 'He is very meagre (?) (*ruqquq*)'. My 'heart' became very 'broken'. Send me a report of your [masc.] illness; .... (BI-*tu-ú ka-lu-ni*)" (AbB 10 28: 7–12). "As to your illness which made you sad (lit. "by which your 'heart' became diseased") and (about which) you wrote to me" (AbB 3 27: 5–6); further on, "the report of your illness" (ibid. 6). If we take the phrase literally, "by which your 'heart' became diseased" (*ša libbaka* [*imr*]*aṣu*), we assume that it be a disease of the belly. A woman writes: "After I had heard of your illness, I became very worried and I am crying the whole day and night" (AbB 7 62: 7–10). A woman in the cloister writes: "I always pray before my Lord and my Mistress for your health. I heard of your illness and I was worried" (AbB 11 106: 3–5).

Two Mari letters speak of the king and a prince being "very ill" (*sul-lu'*).[19]

---

[17] M. Stol, *Birth in Babylonia and the Bible: Its Mediterranean Setting*, Cuneiform Monographs 14 (Groningen: Styx Publications, 2000), 174; E. Leichty, "Feet of Clay," in *DUMU E₂-DUB-BA-A: Studies in Honor of Å.W. Sjöberg*, eds. H. Behrens, D. Loding and M. Roth, Occasional Publications of the Samuel Noah Kramer Fund 11 (Philadelphia: Babylonian Section, University Museum, 1989), 353; M.T. Roth, "Reading Mesopotamian Law Cases: PBS 5 100: A Question of Filiation", *Journal of the Economic and Social History of the Orient* 44 (2001): 258, with explanation, "her worrying threatened her pregnancy and well-being", 272); C. Wilcke in: E.W. Müller, "Familiengründung im Alten Babylonien", in *Geschlechtsreife und Legitimation zur Zeugung*, ed. E.W. Müller, Historische Anthropologie 3 (Freiburg/Munich: J. Martin, Th. Nipperdey, 1985), 278.

[18] ABRT 1 4 III 3–5, with duplicates (W.G. Lambert); see CAD S 96b and the new edition by W.G. Lambert, *Babylonian Oracle Questions*, 90, no. 12c: 11–13.

[19] AEM 1/2 (1988) 425, no. 489: 19, 25 ("Išme-Dagan is not able to come; he is ill (*sú-ul-lu-uḫ*)". We know that he will soon die; S. Lackenbacher, 408; D. Charpin,

The Later Medical Tradition

We translate *salā'u* as "to be ill", *sili'tu* as "illness". The illness *sili'tu* is long-lasting.

- In a ritual from Boghazköy against the fever *li'bu*: "His illness lasted long (*arāku* Dt) and made him bedridden (?) (*nadû*)".[20]
- "If he sees a sheep: (that man): his illness (*si-li-ti-šú*) will last long (GÍD.DA)".[21]
- "If a fit of epilepsy (*miqtu*) befell a baby and it recovered: its illness will last long and it will die".[22] It is possible that death follows ultimately because the cause of the fit is supernatural.

In the poem of the Righteous Sufferer, the patient at first complains "Moreover, my illness has become long" (II 90), and further on: "The conjurer did not clarify the nature of my disease (*šikin murṣija*), nor did the diviner give a time indication (*adannu*) of my illness" (II 110f.). This means that the illness is long but comes to an end at a certain moment (*adannu*), foreseen by the diviner in extispicy. Elsewhere in this poem, the disease is quickly over (*murṣī arḫiš iggamir*) and "in illness ... were long (?)" (*ina si-li-tu i(?)-ri-ku*) (III 48–49).[23]

A physiognomic text, speaking of the fingers of a woman, ends with the unique phrase "illness of the nail" (LÍL UMBIN, *sili'ti ṣupri*): "If she has the illness of the nail, she is lucky".[24] Whatever it means, this must be a chronic ailment.

---

155); M. 7595: 4, cited by D. Charpin, et N. Ziegler, *Mari et le Proche-Orient à l'époque amorrite: essai d'histoire politique*, Florilegium marianum V, Mémoires de N.A.B.U. 6 (Paris: SEPOA, 2003), 137, note 501 ("Le roi [Samsi-Addu] est très malade").

[20] G. Meier, "Ein akkadisches Heilungsritual aus Bogazköy," *Zeitschrift für Assyriologie* 45 (1939): 208 V 20.

[21] TDP 4: 29, with A.R. George, "Babylonian texts from the folios of Sidney Smith. Part two: Prognostic and diagnostic omens, tablet I", *Revue d'Assyriologie* 85 (1991): 144, 164: 28.

[22] TDP 222: 49. J. Scurlock and B.R. Andersen, *Diagnoses in Assyrian and Babylonian Medicine. Ancient Sources, Translations, and Modern Medical Analyses* (Urbana/Chicago: University of Illinois Press, 2005), 316, § 13.176, "(if) his illness is prolonged, he will die".

[23] See for these passages W.G. Lambert, *Babylonian Wisdom Literature* (Oxford: Clarendon Press, 1960), 44, 50.

[24] SpbTU IV 149 II 35; B. Böck, *Die babylonisch-assyrische Morphoskopie*, Archiv für Orientforschung, Beiheft 27 (Vienna: Institut für Orientalistik der Universität, 2000), 158: 142.

The words "for the illness of impotence" (*ana* LÍL ŠÀ.ZI.GA) (in broken context) may refer to a lasting problem.[25]

The following may be a list of chronic diseases: "Concerning disease of the limbs of a man (GIG *minâti* LÚ), illness of the body (*si-li-ti zum-ri*), [wasting] of the flesh ([*šiḫḫa*]*t šīri*), madness (*šinīt ṭēmi*)".[26]

In the omen series *Šumma ālu* we see the sequence: "That man, his days will be short, ...," and "That man will be ill" (*is-sal-l*[*a-'*]) (CT 41 18: 1–3). We observe the opposition "short time" – "long disease" in another forecast: "His days will be short, he will be ill (*is-sal-la-'*)".[27]

The disease lasts more than one day, as in the following examples:

- "That patient will be ill (LÍL) with an illness (*ina* LÍL-*ti*) of two, three days and he will recover."[28]
- "He will be ill (LÍL) with an illness (caused by) sun-heat (LÍL-*ti* UD.DA), two, three days, and he will recover."[29]
- "A disease (GIG, *murṣu*) of one day, an illness (*si-li-ti*) of two days seizes her and she recovers again" (an oracle, *tamītu*).[30]
- "If he is ill (LÍL-*ma*) (for) six days and does not breathe freely (*napāšu*) on the seventh day". A test is done by sprinkling water over his face and his behaviour (whether or not he opens his eyes and cries) will determine the prognosis.[31] This passage suggests that normally the *sili'tu* illness is followed by breathing freely, in other words: recovery.
- "If a man: illness (*si-li-'-tum*) begins on day ..., [and] on ⟨day⟩ 27 blood flows from his mouth (?) ... on day 28 in month VI ....: sorcery has been

[25] G. Beckman and B.R. Foster, "Assyrian Scholarly Texts in the Yale Babylonian Collection", in *A Scientific Humanist: Studies in Memory of Abraham Sachs*, eds. E. Leichty, M. de J. Ellis, and P. Gerardi, Occasional Publications of the Samuel Noah Kramer Fund 9 (Philadelphia: The University Museum, 1988), 12 no. 9b rev. 4.

[26] CT 51 200: 6–7, with collation; W. von Soden, "Review of: The Assyrian Dictionary of the Oriental Institute of the University of Chicago Editorial Board J.A. Brinkman and al. (Eds) vol. 15," *Orientalistische Literaturzeitung* 82 (1987): 459.

[27] F.R. Kraus, *Texte zur babylonischen Physiognomatik*, Archiv für Orientforschung, Beiheft 3, Berlin: Im Selbstverlage des Herausgebers, 1939) text 2b: 9, now B. Böck, *Die babylonisch-assyrische Morphoskopie*, Archiv für Orientforschung 27 (Vienna: Institut für Orientalistik der Universität, 2000), 78: 80.

[28] TDP 156: 3; Heeßel, *Diagnostik*, 195 XVII: 3.

[29] TDP 156: 9; Heeßel, *Diagnostik*, 195 XVII: 9.

[30] K.8139 rev. 11, cited CAD S 263 f, see the new edition by W.G. Lambert, *Babylonian Oracle Questions*, 118 no. 21 rev. 12.

[31] TDP 152: 56; Heeßel, *Diagnostik*, 177 XVI: 63. Scurlock, Andersen, *Diagnoses*, 342, § 13.286 ("coma test"). The passage confirms that *salā'u* and *salāḫu* are variant spellings of one and the same verb: "They will sprinkle (MS F *i-sal-la-ú-ma*, MS H [*i-s*]*al-la-ú*) water onto his face, and ... if he opens and closes his eyes, (and) cries because of the water which they sprinkled (MSS F and H *is-lu-hu-šú*) onto his face, he will recover."

performed against him (*ipšū epšūšu*). Within five days or within .... d[ays] ...: that man will die of an illness (due to) (?) the Hand of Throat-Cutting (LÍL(?)-*ti* ŠU ZI.KU$_5$.RU.DA BAD)".[32]

- In a description of malaria (*di'u*): "The malaria (*di-ḫu*) begins in his body, he gets illness of the belly (LÍL-*ti* ŠÀ *ir-ta-ši*), his bowels void". Its cause is "touch by sun-heat". At the end of this description we read: "That disease is an illness of one day".[33]

"That disease is an illness of one day" does not fit my theory that *sili'tu* is a protracted disease. But there is a solution when we compare this entry (100–105) with the preceding one, which describes the development of malaria during ten days (95–99). Does our entry speak of the same protracted disease, here limited to one day?[34]

R. Labat diagnosed *di'u* as malaria ("Sumpffieber", "paludisme"); here in its first phase; according to him, lines 4–7 of this Tablet XVII describe its second phase.[35]

J. Scurlock and B.R. Andersen diagnose both entries differently. They interpret the first entry (95–99) as describing a patient with an acute infection who develops immunity in the ten days. The second entry (100–105) gets its place in their discussion of the diseases *di'u* and *ṣētu*, with conditions being different, leading to dehydration.[36]

Hemerologies warn: "He should not descend to the garden: he will be ill (*is-sa-la-'*)".[37] Date gardens in Iraq are well watered and the ditches are full of germs. A long disease is possible. Other hemerologies say that one can contract the fever *la'bu* in the lowlands along the canals (*ušallu*).[38]

---

32 STT I 89: 43–47.

33 TDP 168: 100; Heeßel, *Diagnostik*, 205, XVII: 100–103, translated p. 211, comm. p. 216. Scurlock and Andersen (60, 3.164, with p. 602 note 169; cf. Heeßel, 216f.) maintain that the entry in lines 100–103 continues in line 104: "If (it seems to) have finished"; I do not believe this, and side with CAD Q 183b, discussion.

34 Note that the earlier version of lines 95–99 is available and that it is not followed by an entry with the contents of our 100–105. So 100–105 is a later elaboration. See R. Labat, "Une nouvelle tablette de pronostics médicaux", *Syria* 33, (1956): 121: 10–12 and M. Stol, "Fevers in Babylonia," in *Disease in Babylonia*, eds. I.L. Finkel and M.J. Geller, Cuneiform Monographs 36 (Leiden/Boston: Brill, 2007), 16f.

35 R. Labat, "Fieber", *Reallexikon der Assyriologie* 3/1 (1957): 61b; Heeßel, *Diagnostik*, 212 note 7 (on *di'u*), 216 (on 100–105).

36 Scurlock, Andersen, *Diagnoses*, 546, § 20.92 (95–99), 60, 3.164.

37 P. Hulin, "A Hemerological Text from Nimrud," *Iraq* 21 (1959): 50: 37, 52: 46 (= CTN IV 58); also in Assur hemerologies.

38 Hulin, *Iraq* 21 (1959): 52: 47; KAR 177 rev. II 33f., with R. Labat, HMA (1939) 174.

Note that the Diagnostic Handbook once uses the word "a long disease" (GIG GÍD.DA, *murṣu arku*), in: "If he is sick with a long disease". In this passage, he sees things "like" animals, persons, mountains, etc.[39] That diseases last long (*arāku*) is often said in medical texts,[40] but "long disease" is not a technical term.

A Disease of Babies (šerru)

A baby seems to have *sili'tu* illness according to an Old Babylonian letter.[41]

More problematic are two passages in the chapter in the Diagnostic Handbook dealing with babies.

- "If the baby is constantly ill (*ittanasla'*) and, when you pour water on its belly, it does not raise (?) (*elû* Š) its belly: its belly is broken" (TDP 218: 13).[42]
- "If the baby, at the breast of its mother, is restless, is constantly ill (LÍL.LÍL-'); ditto, it cries and fever seizes it all the time: (unfulfilled) vows have seized it" (TDP 220: 20).[43]
- "If a baby constantly turns over (*ittanasḫur*), is constantly ill (*it-ta-na-as-la-'*): Hand of [...]" (TDP 226: 82).[44] In the preceding entry, the baby is *ruššud* (=?), in the next entry he is restless.

Here, we do not expect a long disease but a specific behaviour or symptom, perhaps a symptom close to the literal meaning of the verb, "to sprinkle".

The Old Babylonian List of Diseases, in the section of diseases of the belly, offers: "My belly is ill", šà.mu al.líl = *libbī sà-li-iḫ*.[45] Between *miqit irrim* "collapse of the entrails", and *libbī ītanalliam* "my belly is continually coming up (to vomit)".

---

[39] TDP 196: 58–79; Heeßel, *Diagnostik*, 310–312 XVIII: 22–43.

[40] CAD A/2 224b (3′); M/2 225b. Rituals to prevent the disease *ḫimiṭ ṣēti* from becoming long: Heeßel, *Diagnostik*, 342, XXXI: 4, 7, etc.

[41] A. 138 rev. 1, cited CAD S 96 (*is-sà-li-iḫ-ma*), rev. 4–5, cited CAD Š/2 318a (*a-bi še-er-ri ki-a-am i-ip-pé-eš*) (tablet in the Oriental Institute, Chicago).

[42] Scurlock, Andersen, *Diagnoses*, 416, § 17.164 "If an infant is continually ill and (if) you pour water onto his abdomen, it does not pool (?) in his abdomen, his abdomen has been seriously injured". "To pool" (*šêlu* D) does not exist in Akkadian.

[43] Scurlock, Andersen, *Diagnoses*, 518, § 19.357.

[44] Scurlock, Andersen, *Diagnoses*, 509 f., § 19.319: "If an infant is repeatedly (*ittanasḫur*) (and) continually sick, "hand" of [Gula]". They identify the disease as *kala-azar*.

[45] MSL 9 (1969) 80: 171.

Disease (murṣu) *is Sometimes Opposed to Illness* (sili'tum)

In the omen series *Šumma ālu* we read: "If in month I, between day 1 and day 30, a snake sees a man in the street: either he will be sick (GIG, *imarraṣ*), or he will be ill (*is-sal-la-ʾ-ma*) and he will die".[46] A later commentary no more understood the difference and explained *issallaʾ* as *imarruṣ*.[47]

In the Diagnostic Handbook, there is a passage that discusses new symptoms appearing "in/during his disease" (*ina* GIG-*šú*) (TDP 158: 14–31; Heeßel, Diagnostik 196 XVII: 14–31). In contrast, a few passages speak of "in/during his illness".[48] A tablet with abstracts of prescriptions discusses what happens when "in his illness" (*ina* LÍL-*šú*, variant *si-li-ʾ-ti-šú*) fever (*ummu*) spreads (*epēšu*) to other parts of the body: his head, eyes, ears, neck, belly, lower abdomen (*emšu*), hips, penis, feet (BAM 1 3 III 42-IV 11).[49] In the case of the head and the eyes, the fever will leave (*elû* Gt) that part of the body. In the entry that precedes this section, we read "If a man is diseased (GIG, *maruṣ*) and his disease (*murṣu*) spreads to his head" (III 37).

The passage on the ears deserves our attention. In the original text from which this passage was copied, we see the context. It seems to describe three subsequent cases and treatments.[50]

- "If a man is diseased and his disease expands to the inside of his ears and he is 'heavy' with regard to hearing (i.e. has difficulty hearing)" (BAM 5 503 II 54, dupl. R. Labat, RSO 32 [1957] 114 II 14). During the treatment, pus comes out and is cleaned away (*kapāru*, *gamāru*) and powder is blown into his ear. Recovery is not (yet) promised (II 56–57).

---

[46] CT 38 33: 16, with S.M. Freedman, "BM 129092, A Commentary on Snake Omens," in *If a Man Builds a Joyful House: Assyriological Studies in Honor of of Erle Verdun Leichty*, eds. A.K. Guinan, M. de J. Ellis, A.J. Ferrara, Cuneiform Monographs 31 (Leiden/London: Brill, 2006), 156, "Tablet 22 omen 16".

[47] Freedman, in: *Studies Erle Verdun Leichty* (2006), 150: 8.

[48] I have considered interpreting *i-na*-KID in BAM 5 494 I 35 as *i-na* LÍL, but the suffix -*šú* is not there. CAD R 207a and F. Köcher, "Ein Text medizinischen Inhalts aus dem neubabylonischen Grab 405," in *Uruk; Die Gräber*, eds. R.M. Boehmer et al., Ausgrabungen in Uruk-Warka, 10 (Mainz: Philipp von Zabern, 1995), 211b, read *i-na*-KID (= ?). Scurlock, Andersen, *Diagnoses*, 63, § 3.174, read *i-na-saḫ* "it retracts", a meaning not attested in CAD N/2.

[49] M. Worthington, "Edition of BAM 3," *Le Journal des Médecines Cunéiformes* 7 (2006): 24, 30 f.

[50] BAM 5 503 II 54–62. II 54–57 can be restored thanks to AO. 6774 II 14–20; R. Labat, "Remèdes assyriens contre les affections de l'oreille, d'après un inédit du Louvre (AO. 6774)," *Rivista degli Studi Orientali* 32 (1957): 114.

- "If a man: fever expands to the inside of his ears and his hearing is 'heavy', or he holds sweat" (II 58).[51] The treatment promises: "His hearing will be opened" (*nešmûšu ippette*) (II 60). A diet prescription follows.
- "If a man: in his illness (*ina sili'tišu*) fever expands to the inside of his ears and his ears are 'heavy'" (II 61). The treatment promises: "His hearing will 'lighten'" (*nešmûšu iqallil*). In the end, he will recover (*ina*-[*eš*]) (II 62).

The last passage refers to the last phase of a protracted disease (= *sili'tu*?). Here, the hearing is no more 'heavy'; quite the reverse, it is 'light' again. The patient recovers.

Another fragmentary text speaks of "heavy hearing" in this way: "[...] his [h]earing is 'heavy', in his illness his neck [...]".[52]

Basically, "illness" is not serious. Many omina show that one can recover from it. A Middle-Babylonian omen text from Elam says "[A *si-l*]*i-'-tu* that cannot be removed (*šà* NU *nansuḫi*) will seize a man and he will recover (TI.LA)".[53]

A man "eats bread, drinks beer and chokes (?) and his head is spinning". He is diagnosed as "ill of a gall disease". A potion is prepared and the prescription ends thus: "He will drink (it) on an empty stomach and if it affects him (*ilappatsuma*), he will be ill (*is-sal-la-'*). Do not worry (*la tanakkud*); he will recover. Make him drink it on a propitious day".[54] These lines are unique in the medical corpus. "To affect", literally "to touch" (*lapātu*), always has a negative connotation. I take it to be conditional ("if it affects him"): the patient may experience some setbacks, it may take some time (*salā'u*), but he will recover. Administrating the potion on a propitious day may help.

---

[51] Scurlock, Andersen, *Diagnoses*, 204, 9.104 (under Otitis media), with p. 716 note 127 (parallels).

[52] TDP 126 III 37 (Tablet XIII). The source is LKU 102: 5. There is no basis for *maqissu* at the end of this line; thus TDP, followed by CAD S 263b.

[53] R. Labat avec la collaboration de D.O. Edzard, *Textes Littéraires de Suse*, Mémoires de la Délégation Archéologique en Iran 57. Mission de Susiane. Suse Ville Royale vol. 11 (Paris: Librairie Orientaliste Paul Geuthner, 1974), 97 no. 4 rev. 50, cf. 48.

[54] BAM 6 578 I 41, dupl. BAM 2 159 I 36–37. CAD N/1 153b: "He drinks the medication, if it affects him adversely and he becomes ill, do not worry, he will get well". D. Cadelli, "Recherche sur la Médecine Mésopotamienne, La Série šumma amêlu suâlam maruṣ" (Doctorat de l'Université de Paris I Panthéon Sorbonne, non publiée, 2000), 190, 227: "Si (la potion) devait lui faire beaucoup d'effet et que son état s'aggrave". J. Scurlock, *Magico-Medical Means of Treating Ghost-Induced Illnesses in Ancient Mesopotamia*, Ancient Magic and Divination 3 (Leiden/Boston: Brill-Styx, 2006), 71 follows CAD N/1.

A Diagnosis May be Based on the Etymology of salḫu--salā'u

"If his ears are damp (*sal'ā*) like the ears of a young goat: Hand of a Ghost; in (?) three days he will get a *nikittu*; variant: an illness (LÍL TUKU, *sili'ta iraššši*)" (TDP 70: 16). After the first forecast (*nikittu*) the author added the variant forecast *sili'tu*, perhaps by an association of this word with the "damp" ears (*sal'u*). Cf. the equation *ša-liḫ-tum* = *mas-la-'-tum* "laceration means epidemic" in an extispicy commentary, using the same principle.[55] Moreover, a commentary twice identifies *salā'u* IV with *nakādu* (see below). The word *nikittu* is derived from that verb. That word has been translated as "crisis" and the first meaning of the verb *salā'u* given in *CAD* is "to become ill, to enter the critical stage of an illness" (which is not the same!). This interpretation by *CAD* "to enter the critical stage of an illness" may be based on this commentary, which is demonstrably faulty (see below).[56]

Other Passages

What the conjurer sees on his way to the patient is relevant for the latter. We read in Tablet I of the Diagnostic Handbook:

- "If he stubs the thumb of his right hand: that patient will die within seven days. If he stubs the thumb of his left hand: the patient will be ill (*is-sal-la-'*) and will die; variant: will recover" (TDP 2: 4–5).[57]

The "illness" associated with the left side must last longer than the seven days associated with the right side.

- "If a donkey passes by at his right hand: that diseased person will recover and within one year he will die. If a donkey passes by at his left hand: that diseased person will become ill (LÍL-*ma*) and he will die. Variant: he will recover" (TDP 4: 22 f.).[58]

---

[55] U.S. Koch, *Secrets of Extispicy: The Chapter Multābiltu of the Babylonian Extispicy Series and Niṣirti Bārûti Texts, Mainly from Aššurbanipal's Library*, Alter Orient und Altes Testament 326 (Münster: Ugarit Verlag, 2005), 97 f., line 39. CAD Š/1 244b: meaning uncertain.

[56] As to the young goat and the Hand of a Ghost: Ghosts are associated with goats. J. Scurlock, *Magico-Medical Means of Treating Ghost-Induced Illnesses in Ancient Mesopotamia*, AMD 3 (2006) 101 note 240.

[57] A.R. George, *RA* 85 (1991): 144, 164: 42–43.

[58] Complete in George, *RA* 85 (1991): 142, 164: 20 f.

Both omens associate "illness" with the left side and leave the option of recovery open.

- "If he sees a blind man: he will be sick with a severe disease (GIG *dannu* GIG), he will be ill (LÍL), he will die" (TDP 6: 43).[59] Can we say that blindness, too, is a severe disease that can last long (*salā'u*?), and death follows?
- "If his inner thighs are displaced (*nabalkutu*): his disease will change (for the worse) (*šanû*). If his inner thighs are displaced and the character (UMUŠ, *ṭēmu*) of his illness changes (*nakāru*) for him: Hand of Šamaš; he will recover" (TDP 132 I 63–64).[60] The commentary transposes the Sumerograms for "the character of his illness changes" into Akkadian: *ṭè-eme si-li-ti-šú* KÚR-*ir*.[61] Note that normally a disease has a "nature" (*šiknu*), not a "character" (*ṭēmu*).

The Verb salā'u *in Commentaries*

A commentary on the Diagnostic Handbook comments twice on an Ntn form of *salā'u*, *it-ta-na-as-la-'*. Firstly: [*it*]-*ta-na-as-la-'-ma*: *sa-la-a*$_4$ (A.AN) = *na-ka-da* (8) [x x] x = *ina-an-ziq*;[62] secondly, [LÍL.LÍL-*a'*: *i*]*t-ta-na-as-la-'* = *i-nak-kud* "he worries".[63] This chapter in the Diagnostic Handbook (XL) discusses babies and a "worrying" baby gives no sense. Clearly, "to worry" as an explanation is a guess.

A semantically similar guess is found in the next commentary text:

"If a woman gives birth to a boy cripple (*akû*), the house of the man will be worried (*ultaššaš*)".[64] The last word is commented upon: *ul-ta-aš-šá-aš* = *is-sal-la-'*. The next line explains *issalla'* = *imarraṣ* "he will be ill" - another commentary offers the same explanation.[65] Clearly, at this

[59] Complete in George, *RA* 85 (1991): 144, 164: 34.

[60] Now M.J. Geller, *Renal and Rectal Disease Texts*, Die babylonisch-assyrische Medizin in Texten und Untersuchungen 7 (Berlin/New York: Walter de Gruyter, 2005), 248 no. 49 I 17–18. Cancel in line 18 the "hun.gá-*šú* tag$_4$-*šú*". The copy is Labat, TDP II Pl. XXXVI, K. 3826: 3. Scurlock, Andersen, *Diagnoses*, 495, 19.272: "If his inguinal regions shift constantly under him", in a discussion of the Hand of Šamaš.

[61] SpbTU I 36: 13. No translation in CAD N/1 164a.

[62] SpbTU I 41: 7–8, commentary on TDP 218: 13.

[63] SpbTU I 41: 10, commentary on TDP 220: 20 (correct CAD N/1 153a). Line 9 comments on TDP 218: 16–19 (sorcery).

[64] E. Leichty, *The Omen Series Šumma Izbu*, Texts from Cuneiform Sources 4 (New York: J.J. Augustin, 1970), 36 I: 56.

[65] Leichty, *The Omen Series Šumma Izbu*, Texts from Cuneiform Sources 4 (New York: J.J. Augustin, 1970), 213: 26–27. The other commentary was mentioned above; S.M. Freedman "BM 129092, A Commentary on Snake Omens," in *If a Man Builds a*

time the verb *salā'u* was a difficult word and needed an explanation. An older commentary may have understood its meaning and wished to tell the reader that a (lasting) "illness" meant worries (*nakādu*) in the family. We have seen above that seeing a blind man led to this "illness" and we suggested that both have in common their chronic condition. Here, we can say the same of the cripple that is born: the family will suffer from a chronic worrying = "illness".

A commentary in an astrological handbook reads as follows:

"The king will be ill (*is-sal-la-'*)".[66] Astrology in this handbook always has an effect on the community, not the individual, which is why a public figure, "the king", is here the patient. The commentary reads: *i-sal-la-a'* = *i-ḫar-ra-aṣ*, and continues *aš-šum e-li-tum: ḫar x* [...].[67] This means nothing and one can suspect an error: *iḫarraṣ* ought to be *imarraṣ*.

Excursus on nakādu, nakud, naḫid, na'id

More than once, *salā'u* is equated with *nakādu*, and an excursus on this verb may be in order. W. von Soden, *AHw*, distinguishes between *nakādu* and *naqādu*; *CAD* takes them together under *nakādu*. Von Soden in his review of *CAD N* holds fast to his distinction.[68] The remarkable fact is that with his second verb *naqādu* only the stative is attested. This makes one suspicious: an independent verb with only one form? A late commentary equates *na-'-id* with *na-kud*.[69] This leads us to the verb *na'ādu*. *CAD* has the stative forms *naḫid* and *na'id* (said of a patient) under *na'ādu*, and the form *nakud* (variant *nakid*) under *nakādu*. *AHw* lists the forms *naqid* and *naqud* under his second verb *naqādu*. All these words mean "there is cause for worry", "its is critical". Let me make an attempt at a solution.

Joyful House: Assyriological Studies in Honor of of Erle Verdun Leichty, eds. A.K. Guinan, M. de J. Ellis, A.J. Ferrara, Cuneiform Monographs 31 (Leiden/London: Brill, 2006), 150: 8 (here *imarruṣ*).

66 ACh Second Suppl. 2: 17; now L. Verderame, *Le tavole I–VI della serie astrologica Enūma Anu Enlil*, NISABA 2 (Messina: Dipartimento di scienze dell'antichità, Università di Messina, 2002), 28 I § 19.

67 Verderame *op. cit.* 39 i II 14–15 (cf. 48 t: 8). Copy: E.F. Weidner, "Die astrologische Serie Enûma Anu Enlil," *Archiv für Orientforschung* 14 (1941–1944) Pl. IV (after p. 176).

68 W. von Soden, "Review of: The Assyrian Dictionary of the Oriental Institute of the University of Chicago, eds. J.A. Brinkman et al. Vol 11. Part I and II: N," *Orientalistische Literaturzeitung* 79 (1984): 32 ad S. 153 f.

69 SpbTU I 29 rev. 9.

The forms *naḫid* and *na'id* are variant spellings of the stative of the verb *na'ādu*, a verb of which the G stem is attested in the Old Babylonian period only; later on, forms with the infix *-t-* are used. The two forms *naḫid* and *na'id* continued to be used as frozen forms in the technical language of the Diagnostic Handbook (interestingly not, on current evidence, in the therapeutic corpus).

How can we explain the stative form *naqid*? The adjective *naqdu* occurs in the phrase *marṣu naqdu* "der besorgniserregende Kranke".[70] The present form *inaqqid* of the verb *naqādu* also occurs, "If (the disease) *samānu* afflicts a man's head and it itches and (now) he comes into a worrying state (*i-na-qid*), (now) he comes to rest (*i-na-aḫ*)".[71]

It seems best to interpret the putative verb *naqādu* (with its verbal adjective *naqdu*) as a by-form of the verb *nakādu*, as in *CAD*. Variations in verbal theme vowel (*i/i* vs. *u/u*) are attested in Akkadian. The verb *nakādu* primarily refers to heart-beat and the substantives *nakuttu*, *nikittu* (distinguished by *CAD*) are primarily the pounding of the heart. Often the verb and the substantives function as metaphors for worries and fear. We do not need *niqittu* I "kritischer Zustand, Mühe" in *AHw*. The stative *nakud* of this verb has a meaning so similar to *naḫid* and *na'id* that people saw no difference. A late commentary equates *na-'-id* with *nakud* (see above), which suggests that *na'id* is archaic and little understood. The word *nakud* may have been adopted in medical terminology later.

More Attestations of the Verb salā'u:

- "A lizard will climb onto a person's chair: he will be ill (*is-sa-la-'*)".[72]
- "If a man dreams that 'oil of a wolf' is given to him": "the seizing of illness" (*ṣa-bat si-li-'-ti*) is the forecast. A medical text speaks of "the seizing of (by) a wolf".[73] Can we see a connection?

---

[70] Thus W.R. Mayer, "Das Gebet des Eingeweideschauers an Ninurta," *Or NS* 74 (2005): 52: 5. CAD s.v. *nakdu* "critical, critically ill"; AHw s.v. *naqdu* "dessen Zustand kritisch ist". A commentary on a medical omen is interesting. The omen says that a patient who saw a red pig will die within three months; alternative: three days. The commentary explains: "If he is critically ill (*ki-i na-aq-du*), within three days; if he is not critically ill, within three months he will die"; A.R. George, RA 85 (1991): 148: 8, c. Both alternatives (critical, or not) also in extispicy; U.S. Koch, *Secrets of Extispicy*, 600 s.v. *nakdu*.

[71] BAM 5 494 I 35. See also footnote 48.

[72] KAR 382 rev. 22, dupl. STT II 323: 20. S.M. Moren, Dissertation (1978) 281.

[73] A.L. Oppenheim, *The Interpretation of Dreams in the Ancient Near East. With a Translation of an Assyrian Dream-Book*, Transactions of the American Philosophical

- "If he eats clay (in his dream), he will be restless, he will be ill (LÙ *is-sa-la-'*)".[74]
- "If he eats dust (in his dream), he will be ill (LÍL-*a*), he makes promises (lit. "he talks") but is negligent (?)".[75]

Difficult:

> *šum-ma* É.MEŠ EN LÍL *i-qat-tu-ú* EN.TE.NA RI-*šum-ma*, "(that sick person:) if it is summer, until the illness stops; coldness / winter, will ... upon him and (he will not recover)".[76]

In BAM 6 578 I 30: NA.BI ZÉ LÍL SÌG-*su*. D. Cadelli, Thèse (2000) 189 note 11, 226 reads: ZÉ *saḫ-pa-su*, "cet homme (présente) une vésicule biliaire (qui) est renversée".

sili'tu *in Literary Texts*

In literary texts, *sili'tu* seems to be no more that a variant of *murṣu* "disease". Like the latter, it can be removed (*nasāḫu*). "May Adad decree (*amû* Gt) the removal of illness from my body".[77] "Let the absence of my disease (*la bašê murṣija*), the removal of my illness (*nasāḫ sil'itija*) be on your lips".[78] "May Gula put in his body a never ending disease, a never resting disease, a ... illness".[79]

In the later lexical tradition, they follow each other: [.... TU].RA (?) = *mur-*[*ṣ*]*u*, LÍL = *si-l*[*i-tu*]*m*.[80]

Society 46 (Philadelphia: American Philosophical Society, 1956), 325 x + 21, with p. 279b; the medical text is AMT 61,1: 12 = BAM 7 50 no. 2a: 12. CAD B 108b and Ṣ 164a suggested for the "seizing by a wolf" lycanthropy as interpretation.

[74] A.L. Oppenheim, *The interpretation of Dreams in the Ancient Near East* (1956) 317 y + 6. Oppenheim, *ibidem*: he eats wind (IM). Wrong.

[75] Oppenheim, *op. cit.* 317 y + 10; cf. CAD M/2 8 (*makû*).

[76] TDP 184: 20; far better is Heeßel, *Diagnostik*, 257 XXII: 70. I read at the beginning *šum-ma*, "if (it is summer)", as do Scurlock, Andersen, *Diagnoses* 17, 2.8.

[77] J.V. Kinnier Wilson, "The Kurba'il Statue of Salmaneser III," *Iraq* 24 (1962): 95: 40 = RIMA 3 (1996), 61 no. 12: 40 (Shalmaneser III). The wish of a long life preceeds.

[78] H. Hunger, *Babylonische und assyrische Kolophone*, Alter Orient und Altes Testament 2 (Neukirchen-Vluyn: Verlag Butzon & Bercker Kevelaer, 1968) no. 339: 5, with R. Borger, "Note 8", *Revue d'Assyriologie* 64 (1970): 188.

[79] K. Al-Adami, "A new Kudurru of Marduk-nadin.ahhe: IM. 90585," *Sumer* 38 (1982): 126 VI 9–10; K. Watanabe, *Die adê-Vereidigung anlässlich der Thronfolgeregelung Asarhaddons*, Baghdader Mitteilungen, Beiheft 3 (Berlin: Gebg. Mann Verlag, 1987) 40, below.

[80] STT II 398 I 7–8.

masla'tu, sil'u

The word *masla'tu* is attested only in extispicy forecasts. It always refers to "troops" (erén), either "ours" or those of the enemy.[81] Commentaries equate the word with *šertu* "punishment",[82] and one adds "disease of the belly/heart" (*mas-la-tum* = *mur-ṣu* Š[À]).[83] "Epidemic" has been suggested.

The word *sil'u* means "micturation" according to *CDA*. This is based on the context, "When his 'sprinkling' has soiled him (*lapātu*)".[84]

The Sumerogram líl literally means "wind", which can be a cause of disease. "Winds of the desert will often have caused illness".[85]

I thank Martin Worthington for his critical and invaluable assistance.

---

[81] U. Koch-Westenholz, *The Babylonian Liver Omens: The Chapters Manzāzu, Padānu and Pān Tākalti of the Babylonian Extispicy Series, Mainly from Aššurbanipals's Library*, CNI Publication 25 (Copenhagen: Carsten Niebuhr Institute Publications, 2000), 514, Index of words, s.v. ("a disease").

[82] TBP 25: 2, Böck, *Morphoskopie* 288, "Er ist sehr lang. Strafe, Epidemie".

[83] SpbTU I 83 rev. 7; Böck, *Morphoskopie* 255: 43 (Rs. 7).

[84] Geller, BAM 7 58 no. 3 II 8, 29 [so!]. If Geller's *sil'ušu* is correct, we are reminded of *tal'ašu*, "Kornwurm", als Krankheit (AHw).

[85] Th. Jacobsen, "The lil$_2$ of ^{d}En-lil$_2$" in *DUMU-E$_2$-DUB-BA-A: Studies in Honor of Å.W. Sjöberg*, eds. H. Behrens, D. Loding and M. Roth, Occasional Publication of the Samuel Noah Kramer Fund 11 (Philadelphia: Babylonian Section, University Museum, 1989), 271.

SOME NOTES ON MEDICAL INFORMATION OUTSIDE THE MEDICAL CORPORA

Martin Worthington*

To date, discussions of healing in Mesopotamia tend to focus on ancient "professional" medical literature, i.e. on the corpora of medical (therapeutic and diagnostic) tablets. The reasons for this are clear and proper, but at the same time it is important to note that there are significant qualitative limitations to the information which the currently known medical corpora can yield.

Before these limitations are introduced, it is important to recognise that discussants of Mesopotamian healing have repeatedly drawn on non-medical sources, primarily letters. Already in 1965, E. Ritter included a selection of Middle Babylonian and Neo-Assyrian letters of medical interest in her famous article in the *Festschrift* for Benno Landsberger.[1] More recently, illnesses and doctors in Mari were studied by J.-M. Durand on the evidence of letters;[2] L. Sassmannshausen gathered references to doctors in Middle Babylonian administrative

* The bulk of the research for this article was undertaken during a re-invitation scholarship of the German Academic Exchange Service (DAAD) held in Leipzig and Heidelberg from March to May 2006. I am deeply beholden to the DAAD for the opportunity to conduct the research and enjoy interesting and instructive conversations with Dr Nils Heeßel and Prof. Annette Zgoll, who also commented most usefully on drafts of this paper. It is a pleasure further to thank Professors Tzvi Abusch, Andrew George and Marten Stol for their careful scrutiny and very valuable suggestions.

[1] E. Ritter, "Magical-Expert (=*ĀŠIPU*) and Physician (=*ASÛ*). Notes on Two Complementary Professions in Babylonian Medicine" in *Studies in Honor of Benno Landsberger on his Seventy-Fifth Birthday, April 21, 1965*, eds. H.G. Güterbock and T. Jacobsen, Assyriological Studies 16 (Chicago: Oriental Institute; University of Chicago, 1965), 317–321.

[2] J.-M. Durand, "Maladies et médecins", in *Archives Épistolaires de Mari I/1*, Archives Royales de Mari 26/1 (Paris: Editions Recherche sur les Civilisations, 1988), 543–584. See previously C. Jean, "Pharmacopée et parfumerie dans quelques lettres de Mari", *Archiv Orientální* 17/1 (1949): 320–329 and A. Finet, "Les médecins au royaume de Mari", *Annuaire de l'Institut de Philologie et d'Histoires Orientales et Slaves* 14 (1954–1955): 123–144.

documents;[3] W. Farber used Mari letters to investigate beliefs relating to contagion;[4] K. Volk collected letters which mention diseases of children;[5] N.P. Heeßel discussed references to medical diagnosis in non-medical sources;[6] M. Stol made a letter-based study of nutrition and bodily care in Old Babylonian times;[7] P. Villard examined the evidence of letters for healers and healing at the Neo-Assyrian court;[8] M.J. Geller discussed a number of letters in connection with the rationale behind the choice of curative substances.[9] E. Robson presented three investigations of medical matters, drawing on Sumerian literature and Neo-Assyrian scholarly letters.[10] Incidental references to non-medical sources bearing on medical matters are further scattered through many discussions of various aspects of Mesopotamian medicine.[11]

---

[3] L. Sassmannshausen, *Beiträge zur Verwaltung und Gesellschaft Babyloniens in der Kassitenzeit*, Baghdader Forschungen 21 (Mainz: Philipp von Zabern, 2001), 72–73. Note especially the reference to a gal *a-se-e* "chief of the *asûs*", which "vielleicht auf eine hierarchische Gliederung der Ârtzteschaft hin[deutet]" (p. 73 with fn. 1177).

[4] W. Farber, "How to Marry a Disease: Epidemics, Contagion and a Magic Ritual against the 'Hand Of Ghost'," in *Magic and Rationality in Ancient Near Eastern and Graeco-Roman Medicine*, eds. H.F.J. Horstmanshoff and M. Stol, in collaboration with C.R. van Tilburg, Studies in Ancient Medicine 27 (Leiden/Boston: Brill, 2004), 117–132.

[5] K. Volk, "Kinderkrankheiten nach der Darstellung babylonisch-assyrischer Keilschrifttexte," *Orientalia* 68 (1999): 6–10.

[6] N.P. Heeßel, *Babylonisch-assyrische Diagnostik*, Alter Orient und Altes Testament 43 (Münster: Ugarit-Verlag, 2000), 92–94.

[7] D. Charpin, D. Edzard, and M. Stol, *Mesopotamien: Die altbabylonische Zeit*, Orbis Biblicus et Orientalis 160/4 (Freiburg/Göttingen: Vandenhoeck & Ruprecht, 2004), 973–975.

[8] P. Villard, "Les guérisseurs à la cour néo-assyrienne," in *Médecine et médecins au Proche-Orient ancien, Actes du Colloque International organisé à Lyon les 8 et 9 novembre 2002, Maison de l'Orient et de la Méditerranée*, eds. L. Battini and P. Villard, BAR International Series 1528 (Oxford: John and Erika Hedge Ltd, 2006), 139–160.

[9] M.J. Geller, "La médecine au quotidien", *Le Journal des Médecines Cunéiformes* 8 (2006): 2–6.

[10] E. Robson, "Mesopotamian Medicine and Religion: Current Debates, New Perspectives," *Religion Compass* 2/4 (Blackwell, 2008, available from: http://www.blackwell-compass.com/subject/religion/): 464–476.

[11] Note especially M. Stol, "Diagnosis and Therapy in Babylonian Medicine", *Jaarbericht Ex Oriente Lux* 32 (1991–1992): 43–65 and P. Attinger, "La médecine mésopotamienne", *Le Journal des Médecines Cunéiformes* 11–12 (2008): 44–51. M. Stol, "Fevers in Babylonia", in *Disease in Babylonia*, eds. I.L. Finkel and M.J. Geller, Cuneiform Monographs 36 (Leiden/Boston: Brill, 2007), 1–39 uses letters to elucidate descriptions of symptoms on medical tablets. R. Labat, "Ordonnances médicales ou magiques", *Revue d'Assyriologie* 54 (1960): 171 fn. 3, compares a symptom on a medical tablet with the

At the same time, the limitations to the informativeness of the medical corpora have perhaps not yet been sufficiently problematised,[12] and full "dialogue" has not yet been achieved between medical and non-medical sources. One rarely encounters references to non-medical sources in editions of Mesopotamian medical tablets, and more frequent references to medical tablets could prove rewarding in medically oriented discussions of non-medical sources.[13]

This article will first spotlight some of the limitations of the medical corpora (§ 1), then discuss selected aspects of healing about which non-medical sources are informative, sometimes more so than medical

illness of the Elamite king recorded in the Babylonian chronicle. W.G. Lambert, *Babylonian Wisdom Literature* (Oxford: Clarendon Press, 1960), 294 observes apropos of *Ludlul* II 108–111: "This is no literary fiction; an actual case occurs in the letter ABL 391 [now SAA X 315, MW] obv. 7–12". Ph. Abrahami, "À propos des fonctions de l'*asû* et de l'*âšipu*", *Le Journal des Médecines Cunéiformes* 2 (2003): 19–20, observes that hymns to Gula can throw light on the functions of the *asû* (cf. § 5 below). K. van der Toorn, *Sin and Sanction in Israel and Mesopotamia—a comparative study*, Studia Semitica Neerlandica 22 (Assen/Maastricht: van Gorcum, 1985), 78 cites Old Babylonian and Old Assyrian letters illustrating the use of divination in making diagnoses/prognoses. D. Cadelli, "Lorsque l'enfant paraît … malade", *Ktema* 22 (1997): 22 fn. 76, cites an Old Babylonian letter (AbB I 31) about breastfeeding which is similar to a passage in the *Diagnostic Handbook* (*TDP* 220–222: 36–37; JA. Scurlock and B.R. Andersen, *Diagnoses in Assyrian and Babylonian Medicine. Ancient Sources, Translations, and Modern Medical Analyses* (Urbana/Chicago: University of Illinois Press, 2005), 410, § 17.143). N.P. Heeßel, "Der verschwiegene Unterschied: Die Geschlechterdifferenz in medizinischen Texten aus dem Alten Mesopotamien," in *Krankheit und Heilung: Gender—Religion—Medizin*, eds. B. Heininger, R. Lindner, and E. Klinger (Münster: Lit, 2006), 12–13 cites Old Babylonian period ration lists and letters showing that female *asûs* existed, and Neo-Assyrian letters showing that female patients were examined by male physicians. M. Widell, "The Sumerian Expression igi-kar$_2$ Revisited," *Iraq* 70 (2008): 131–145 shows that deliveries of foodstuffs and beer termed 'igi-kar$_2$' in Ur$_3$ administrative documents are often connected with childbirth in prominent families, and so, assuming a very plausible connection with the compound verb igi…kar$_2$ 'to examine', he deduces that newly born children in prominent families were subject to a medical inspection which, if favourable, resulted in festivities.

[12] But see E. Ritter in *Studies Landsberger*, 229–230: "We shall … limit our present investigation to the medical texts called canonical [i.e. the medical corpora, MW], naïvely accepting them at face value, and neglect such tangential considerations as the historical position of *āšipu* and *asû*, legal and poetic references to them, the vast non-medical literature of *āšipūtu*, and the question of whether these texts were in fact the basis for medical practice". (Though actually her article includes a very interesting selection of letters, some of which are cited also in this paper. See fn. 1 above).

[13] The statement by Scurlock and Andersen, *Diagnoses*, xxii that "The quality of medical information contained in ancient letters is of considerably less value than either the therapeutic texts or the diagnostic/prognostic handbook" should be understood as referring to descriptions of disease, and reflects the orientation of their book. For other aspects of Mesopotamian healing, letters are invaluable sources.

ones. We will consider the location of therapy (§ 2), the availability and affordability of healers (§ 3), healers' activities outside healing (§ 4), the role of divination in healing (§ 5), and the composition of prescriptions (§ 6). Cumulatively, it is hoped that the medical corpora's proper place in the overall study of Mesopotamian illness and healing will be discerned with greater clarity, and that students of these topics will be encouraged to make greater and more systematic use of non-medical sources.

Unlike grammar, where the examination of a large number of sources can lead to the formulation of a simple and generally valid rule, studies of ancient healing must reckon with a great complexity and diversity of practice, with differences determined by epoch, place, social class, and other factors. Thus even a small number of sources can produce inconsistent snapshots of ancient procedures. Accordingly, the discussions which follow are not, and could not hope to be, comprehensive or definitive statements. Rather they are offered as tesserae from a large mosaic, much of which still has to be pieced together. As more sources are studied, new tesserae will be found.

1. *Some Limitations to the Informativeness of the Medical Corpora*

There are many aspects of professional healing on which the medical corpora are largely or completely silent.[14] Social issues, including the training and remuneration of practitioners,[15] are one example.[16] Doctor-patient relations,[17] patients' experience of disease, the locus of

[14] Some of these are discussed by M.J. Geller, "Ancient medicine: the patient's perspective," *Journal of Nephrology* 17/4 (2004): 605–610, though we cannot concur with several of the statements made there, e.g. "None of the surviving medical corpus tells us ... whether Mesopotamian healers ever indulged in simple surgery or even blood-letting" (cf. fn. 23 below and Attinger, "La médecine mésopotamienne", 73) and "we have no records of patients paying privately for medical treatment" (cf. § 3, below).

[15] Cf. M.J. Geller, "Review of: Vivian Nutton, Ancient Medicine (Routledge, 2004)", *Bulletin of the School of Oriental and African Studies* 69/3 (2006): 462: "An Assyriologist working on Babylonian medicine is equally jealous of the data from the Graeco-Roman world on how physicians were paid and how they functioned in public and private practice ..., since one lacks this kind of information." (Though see §§ 3–4 below).

[16] On the social standing of *asûs* in Ebla see F. Pomponio, "Considerazioni sul medico eblaita e i suoi strumenti di lavoro", in *Semitic and Assyriological Studies Presented to Pelio Fronzaroli by Pupils and Colleagues*, ed. P. Marrassini (Wiesbaden: Harrassowitz Verlag, 2003), 136–149.

[17] If the word is correctly read (*kīma ša-a[b]*ˀ*-sú-ti-ma*), in AbB X 57: 11 third parties are said to be as mendacious 'as a midwife'. This sort of sentiment is, not surprisingly,

therapy, and the role (if any) of the temple are others.[18] The medical corpora usually neither recognise the existence of epidemics, nor indicate how the state dealt with them.[19] Veterinary prescriptions are extremely rare,[20] even though it is known that animals were treated, and some professionals seem to have specialised in this.[21] Regarding practical aspects of medical therapy, mention of divination is almost absent from the medical corpora though there are external indications it was used in healing,[22] and prescriptions for surgery are surprisingly rare.[23] It is

---

absent from the professional corpora, where midwives are in any case badly underrepresented (see M. Stol, *Birth in Babylonia and the Bible: Its Mediterranean Setting*, Cuneiform Monographs 14 (Groningen: Styx Publications, 2000), 171–192).

[18] H. Avalos, *Illness and health care in the ancient Near East: The role of the temple in Greece, Mesopotamia, and Israel*, Harvard Semitic Museum Monographs 54 (Atlanta: Scholars Press, 1995), 218–219 observed that colophons show tablets with medical content to have been copied from temple libraries. F. Joannès, "Traitement des malades et *bit hilṣi* en Babylonie récente", in *Médecine et médecins*, 73–90, has recently shown that the *bīt ḫilṣi* of several Babylonian temples in the late period was a structure in which pharmaceutical substances were processed. See also M. Stol, *JEOL* 32 (1991–1992): 57 on sanctuaries (*aširtus*).

[19] On epidemics in Mari letters see Durand, *AEM* I/1, 544–549.

[20] An example is BAM 159 v.33–36 (cf. KADP 33 rev.4).

[21] See R.D. Biggs, "Medizin," *Reallexikon der Assyriologie* 7 (1987–1990): 629b (with ref. to passages in *CAD* A/ii 347b and M/ii 199a, especially *Codex Hammurapi* §§ 224 and 225), and Durand, *AEM* I/1, 555. Treatment is sought for a wounded ox in AbB IX 71 and perhaps also VI 152. In AbB XIV 111: 39 sheep are said to have died *ina ḫunnuqi* "through *constriction*", implying that a diagnosis was made (though whether by a specialist or not is impossible to tell). A Sumerian seal belonging to an a.zu who is sukkal of the god Gir (i.e. Šakkan), "who helps mother(-animal)s give birth," depicts instruments similar to those used in modern veterinary gynaecology (see I. Fuhr, "Ein sumerischer Tierarzt," *Archiv Orientální* 34 (1966): 570–573). For Ebla, see P. Fronzaroli, "A Veterinary Prescription Found at Ebla (TM.75.G.1645)," in *Memoriae Igor M. Diakonoff; Babel und Bibel 2: Annual of Ancient Near Eastern, Old Testament, and Semitic Studies*, eds. L. Kogan et al., Orientalia et Classica, Papers of the Institute of Oriental and Classical Studies 8 (Winona Lake, IN: Eisenbrauns, 2005), 89–99 and M.G. Biga, "(Foreign) Veterinarians at Ebla", *Nouvelles Assyriologiques Brèves et Utilitaires*, 2006/4, 85.

[22] See e.g. Durand, *AEM* 1/I, 27 and Stol, *JEOL* 32 (1991–1992): 56–58.

[23] The sources for surgery were discussed by R. Labat, "A propos de la chirurgie babylonienne", *Journal Asiatique* 242 (1954): 207–218. The passage in UGU 1 (lines 190′–97′) has been re-edited in M. Worthington, "Edition of UGU 1 (=*BAM* 480 etc.)", *Le Journal des Médecines Cunéiformes* 5 (2005): 13. On AMT 49,4 see M. Stol "An Assyriologist reads Hippocrates," in *Magic and Rationality*, 71–72. For references to surgical instruments see *CAD s.v. karzillu, quppû, naglabu*, and note R.L. Miller, "Eye surgery and *ṣillu*, 'pterygium, conjunctival degeneration'", *Nouvelles Assyriologiques Brèves et Utilitaires*, 1989/1, 10, on AMT 12,1 and "a small bronze knife (? lancet) with a hooked tip" from Tepe Giyan. On blood letting see Biggs, *RlA* 7, 629a (with ref. to BAM 323: 94–95, now Scurlock, AMD 3

letters, not the medical corpora, which attest to the realisation that disease could be transmitted through the use of an ill person's cup and the like.[24]

Another limitation to the informativeness of the medical corpora is that they are severely laconic about their own logic and *Sitz im Leben*.[25] Therapeutic tablets do not normally specify who chose the curative substances, or on what basis;[26] nor how quantities should be determined by the practitioner when the prescription does not specify them; nor how practitioners were supposed to choose between different prescriptions for the same malady,[27] or between alternative substances in the same prescription.[28] Diagnostic tablets rarely explain the rationale behind the association of a particular illness with a particular deity.[29] Such issues doubtless gave rise in antiquity to a large body of oral explanation and commentary,[30] at present largely lost.[31] This is illustrated by a Neo-Assyrian scholar writing in a letter that the proper way for the king to take a medical potion is to drink three drops diluted in specially

no. 91: 1–7) and M. Stol, "Old Babylonian ophthalmology" in *Reflets des deux fleuves: Volume de mélanges offerts à André Finet*, eds. M. Lebeau and Ph. Talon, Akkadica Supplementa 6 (Leuven: Peeters Publishers, 1989), 163–166.

[24] On contagion see Farber in *Magic and Rationality*, 117–132 and Joannès in *Médecine et médecins*, 143–144.

[25] Cf. Geller, *BSOAS* 69/3 (2006): 461: 'We simply have lists of symptoms with some additional remarks and recipes, but no theoretical discussions of medicine'.

[26] Cf. M.J. Geller, "A Babylonian Perspective on Greek Medicine", *Medical History* 50/3 (2006): 393: "What we have in Mesopotamia is a system of medicine … consisting of long lists of diagnostic symptoms and equally lengthy lists of recipes, without any explanatory theses or treatises explaining how and why these remedies were conceived and developed. The lack of any discussion of theory, however, may simply mean that theory was never recorded in writing".

[27] For an exception see no. 1 in M.J. Geller, *Renal and Rectal Disease Texts*, Die babylonisch-assyrische Medizin in Texten und Untersuchungen 7 (Berlin/New York: Walter de Gruyter, 2005), where it is specified that the prescriptions should be tried sequentially.

[28] See § 6 below.

[29] Such tacit rationales can however be deduced by modern scholars, see Stol, *JEOL* 32 (1991–1992): 44–45 and Heeßel, *Diagnostik*, 58–60.

[30] Cf. Geller, *Medical History* 50/3 (2006): 393: "Whatever survives in writing represents only a small selection of medical texts, some of which must have likewise existed in oral form, and this situation can easily distort any general conclusions we seek to make regarding ancient medicine".

[31] Though written medical commentaries are known, e.g. M. Civil, "Medical Commentaries from Nippur," *JNES* 33 (1974): 329–338 and I.L. Finkel in *Cuneiform Texts in the Metropolitan Museum of Art* II, eds. I. Spar and W.G. Lambert (New York: Metropolitan Museum of Art, 2005), 279–283. Several remain unpublished.

prepared water.[32] The interesting point is that the scholar mentions that this procedure is *kī mašqīt mēmēni* "as (for) any potion": this instruction is not currently known from the therapeutic corpus, and would probably have surprised the original authors of the recipes. The letter thus testifies to a specification which medical recipes had accrued orally by the Neo-Assyrian period, without it entering their written transmission.[33]

A feature of the therapeutic corpus (more than of the diagnostic corpus) is that it is at present poorly susceptible to the study of temporal and geographical variation.[34] Therapeutic tablets are overwhelmingly Neo-Assyrian, and the majority of them derive from a small number of sites (Assur, Kuyunjik, Sultantepe).[35] There is not yet sufficient evidence to undertake systematic identification of local differences and traditions, though there are occasional indications of regional variation.[36] Sumerian

[32] SAA X 336 (as discussed in M. Worthington, "Edition of BAM 3," *Le Journal des Médecines Cunéiformes* 7, (2006): 19, *ad* BAM 3 i.18; however, the second person singular verbal forms render it unlikely that the letter was written to the king, more likely to a colleague; correct *JMC* 7 accordingly). One might wonder whether the number three possesses a ritual significance. A hymn to Gula published by Geller in BAM 7 (no. 9 ii.1′–8′), was to be recited three times when taking a drug ("You know what I do not know. I will drink this drug, through this drug may I be cured").

[33] As noted by Heeßel, *Diagnostik*, 91, in another letter the same scholar quotes verbatim from the medical corpus: cf. SAA X 326: 3′-r.3 with BAM 574 i.30 and 32, SA.GIG 17/100–103. Cf. also below with fn. 111.

[34] On differences in Babylonian and Assyrian diagnostic traditions see N.P. Heeßel in *Assur-Forschungen*, forthcoming (Harrassowitz). (On the exceptional rarity of diagnostic tablets in Assur – none found in the library of the *āšipu* Kiṣir-Aššur – see Stol, *JEOL* 32 (1991–1992): 62 and Heeßel, *Diagnostik*, 109 with fn. 55).

[35] Nonetheless, it should be recognized that Assyrian scribes and scholars would have been able to draw on Babylonian medical writings: the Tukultī-Ninurta epic mentions that TN plundered Babylonian *malṭarāt asûti nēpeš naṣm[adāte* ...] "medical prescriptions, rituals for poul[tices ...]" (W.G. Lambert, "Three Unpublished fragments of the Tukulti-Ninurta Epic," *AfO* 18 (1957): 44: 8). On Assyrians plundering Babylonian tablets see also S. Parpola, "Assyrian Library Records", *JNES* 42/1 (1983): 11.

[36] See I.L. Finkel, "On Late Babylonian Medical Training," in *Wisdom, Gods and Literature. Studies in Assyriology in Honour of W.G. Lambert*, eds. A.R. George and I.L. Finkel (Winona Lake, IN: Eisenbrauns, 2000), 141 and 189, on a medical fragment which, if (with Finkel) restored to resemble the astronomical tablet cited in Finkel's fn. 11 (p. 141), instructs the reader not to teach medicine to anyone from particular towns (including Borsippa and Marda). See also I.L. Finkel, "Magic and Medicine at Meskene," *Nouvelles Assyriologiques Brèves et Utilitaires*, 1999/2, 28–30 n. 30 arguing that the use of ZA for *awīlu* on a medical tablet from Meskene/Emar is suggestive of a local tradition. (ZA for *awīlu* is rare on Mesopotamian medical tablets, though cf. *Studies Lambert* 191: 25 for an attestation in Late Babylonian and D. Schwemer, *Akkadische Rituale aus Hattusa: Die Sammeltafel KBo XXXVI 29 und verwandte Fragmente*, Texte der Hethiter 23 (Heidelberg: Universitätsverlag C. Winter, 1998), 5 fn. 19 on KUB XXXVI 56).

medicine is known to have existed, but documentation for it is scarce,[37] and it is currently difficult to attempt to write a connected history of Mesopotamian healing, even though some developments are known to have taken place,[38] and others doubtless await identification.

Finally, even if the medical corpora were larger, less fragmentary, better distributed across time and space, and less laconic to boot, they would still be overwhelmingly biased towards healing as effected by literate professionals. The question would still stand, as it does all the more in the situation we actually face, to what extent the medical corpora are representative of the variety of healing techniques used by different social classes in Mesopotamia.

---

[37] Extant Sumerian medical writings are at present confined to the tablets published by Civil: M. Civil, "Prescriptions médicales sumériennes", *Revue d'Assyriologie* 54 (1960): 57–72 and M. Civil, "Une nouvelle prescription médicale sumérienne", *RA* 55 (1961): 91–94. However, there is evidence for Sumerian surgery in literary descriptions of Ninisina (Gula) wielding a scalpel (see *PSD* B 176a) and in stipulations of wages for the azu in the Ur-Namma lawcode (C.B.F. Walker and P. Michalowski, "A New Sumerian 'Law Code'", in *DUMU E₂-DUB-BA-A: Studies in Honor of Å.W. Sjöberg*, eds. H. Behrens, D. Loding and M. Roth, Occasional Publication of the Samuel Noah Kramer Fund 11 (Philadelphia: Babylonian Section, University Museum, 1989), 389). Some evidence surrounding Sumerian concerns for hygiene may also be cited: in the *Dispute between Bird and Fish* the bird tells the fish that "He who has carried you does not let his hand touch his body" (lú lah_4-a-zu šu-ni su-ni-šè nu-ub-tag-ge, ETCSL line 62); more generally, one proverb holds that "Putting unwashed hands in one's mouth is disgusting" (B. Alster, *Proverbs of Ancient Sumer: The World's Earliest Proverb Collections* (Bethesda, Maryland: CDL Press, 1997), 3.161) and another that "To serve beer with unwashed hands, to spit without trampling upon it, to sneeze without covering it up with dust, to kiss with the tongue at midday without providing shade, are abominations to Utu" (Alster, *Proverbs*, 3.8). The proverb's sentiment about hand-washing when serving beer finds echo a line in *Enlil and Sud*: "According to her mother's instructions she washed her hands and placed a (beer) tankard in his hand" (ETCSL line 82). On Sumerian veterinary medicine and healing at Ebla see fn. 21. A bilingual Sumerian-Akkadian fragment from Late Babylonian Uruk (SpTU I 86) uses phrases characteristic of the diagnostic corpus (see A. Cavigneaux, "Un texte médical bilingue", *Nouvelles Assyriologiques Brèves et Utilitaires*, 1988, no. 2: 19). See also Fincke in this volume.

[38] N.P. Heeßel, "Stein, Pflanze, und Holz: ein neuer Text zur 'medizinischen Astrologie,'" *Orientalia* 74 (2005): 1–22 and "Diagnosis, Divination and Disease: Towards an Understanding of the *Rationale* behind the Babylonian *Diagnostic Handbook*," in *Magic and Rationality*, 97–116 argues for paradigm shifts in Mesopotamian medicine. See further JA. Scurlock and F.N.H. Al-Rawi, "A Weakness for Hellenism," in *If a Man Builds a Joyful House: Assyriological Studies in Honor of Erle Verdun Leichty*, eds. A.K. Guinan et al., Cuneiform Monographs 31 (Leiden/London: Brill, 2006), 357–382. On the gradual rise of the profile of witchcraft in the therapeutic corpus, documented by text-critical study of recipes, see Tz. Abusch, "Witchcraft and the Anger of the Personal god," in *Mesopotamian Witchcraft: Toward a History and Understanding of Babylonian Witchcraft Beliefs and Literature*, Ancient Magic and Divination 5 (Leiden/Boston/Köln: Brill/Styx, 2002).

We might in this connection cite a passage from Herodotus's description of Babylon:

> **Herodotus, *Histories*, I 197** (translation adapted from that of A.D. Godley)
>
> I come next to the wisest of their customs: having no use for physicians, they carry the sick into the *agora*. Then those who have been afflicted by the same ailment as the sick man's, or seen others in like case, come near and advise him about his disease and comfort him, telling him by what means they have themselves recovered from it or seen others so recover. None may pass by the sick man without speaking and asking what his sickness is.

As observed by many discussants,[39] Herodotus's implication that there were no doctors in Babylon is radically at odds with Mesopotamian evidence, and not credible. This, however, does not necessarily mean that his account is mendacious:[40] it could rather derive from an innocent misinterpretation of something he actually saw. If there were Babylonians who could not afford the services of professional healers, it is not difficult to imagine some of them ending up in public places, begging or even seeking advice on possible cures.[41] Had Herodotus seen such people, he might have obtained the impression that this was the norm for all Babylonians: it is thus possible that he records a Mesopotamian historical reality, distorted through the prism of his own erroneous interpretation.[42] Given their biases towards literate and wealthier social groups, this possibility is consistent with the absence of similar reports from Cuneiform sources. Be that as it may, an interesting feature of Herodotus's report from an Assyriological point of view, regardless of its actual historicity, is that it reminds us of how lacunary our current knowledge of Mesopotamian healing practices actually is.

The full publication of Mesopotamian medical literature is and remains an urgent desideratum, but the point stressed here is that, if a nuanced and fulsome understanding of Mesopotamian healing is ever to be achieved, medical sources will require serious complementation. Sometimes, it is true, detailed studies of the corpora themselves can

---

[39] E.g. recently Joannès in *Médecine et médecins*, 73.

[40] The extent to which Herodotus really travelled (or, if he did travel extensively, the extent to which he embellished his experiences of travel) is a contentious issue.

[41] One supposes beggars on the streets as a matter of course, but corroboration for Old Babylonian times is available e.g. in AbB XIV 164: 7–8 ŠE*'um ul ibašši gamer / ana sūqim lūṣi* "There is no barley. All has been spent! Should I go out into the street (to beg)?"

[42] Since this article was submitted for publication a similar conclusion was reached by Attinger, *La médecine mésopotamienne*, 2–3.

illumine issues on which the corpora are silent. But more generally, it is useful to cast one's net as widely as possible, since much information on topics related to healing can be obtained from sources outside the medical corpora, notably letters. This information not only complements that derived from the medical corpora, but can even act as a corrective to their biases. The following sections will attempt to illustrate its usefulness.

2. *Location*

One of the practical aspects of healing on which the medical corpora contain few explicit statements is location.[43] This is because the majority of treatments prescribed are location-independent. Even when patients' beds are specifically mentioned,[44] there is usually no way of telling whether they are in bed at home or elsewhere.[45] A rare hint within the medical corpora is the beginning of Esagil-kīn-apli's *Diagnostic Handbook*, which runs *enūma ana bīt marṣi āšipu*(ka.pirig) *illaku* 'When the *āšipu* goes to a patient's home', implying that the *āšipu* routinely performed home visits to the sick.

That Mesopotamian healing professionals moved around and visited patients at home is borne out by many sources outside the medical corpora.[46] A well-known example is the comic tale of *The Poor Man of Nippur*,[47] in which the central character, disguised as an *asû*, presents himself at the house of the mayor, whom he has just badly beaten, and offers to cure him: the story implies that this was standard practice.

---

[43] "Location" is used here to signify the type of surroundings (bedroom, river bank, etc.) in which the cure is effected. For the locations of rituals against ghosts see JA. Scurlock, *Magico-Medical Means of Treating Ghost-Induced Illnesses in Ancient Mesopotamia*, Ancient Magic and Divination 3 (Leiden/Boston: Brill-Styx, 2006), 22 with references. For a different example see AMT 88,2: 3 *ana bīti eṭî ša išātu u nūra lā immaru ēribšu* "to a house of darkness where the one who enters it sees no fire or light". Location in the sense of 'region of the country' is a different issue. In the Old Babylonian period Mari seems to have enjoyed prestige (Durand, *AEM* I/1, 599), as Isin also did for longer. Durand questions whether the reputation of such centres stemmed from the skill of human professional healers, or from shrines of highly regarded healing deities.

[44] E.g. LKA 69: r.4, AMT 5,5: 10.

[45] In some cases, seclusion (*bītu parsu*) was imposed. See van der Toorn, *Sin and Sanction*, 75.

[46] The movements of healing professionals require investigation in their own right.

[47] Translated with refs. in B.R. Foster, *Before the Muses: An Anthology of Akkadian Literature* (3rd edition; Bethesda: CDL Press, 2005), 931–936.

Letters also document requests for doctors to be dispatched to patients.[48]

However, other sources from outside the medical corpora suggest that home visits are not the whole story.[49] One example is an Old Babylonian letter:

AbB VIII 95: 7–14 (Bēlī-[...] to Ilšu-naṣir)

anum-ma / é.idim.an.šúm / [x (*ḫ*)*a*]*mmurapi* / [*aṭ*]*ṭardakkum* / *a*[*mu*]*ršu-ma* / *ša arḫiš* / *bulluṭešu* / *epuš*
Herewith [I s]end you E-idim-an-šum, the [... of (H)a]mmurapi. Ex[ami]ne him and do what is necessary to cure him quickly.

amāru (lit. "to see") is the technical term for a medical examination.[50] It seems that a patient was sent to a healer accompanied by a covering letter.

Another case of a patient going to the healer is documented by a Late Babylonian administrative tablet (CT 56, 618) to which attention was recently drawn by F. Joannès.[51] The tablet records that 1 *kurru* of dates was delivered to ᴵ*ba-ku-ú-a šá bīt*(é) *a-se-e*, literally to "Bakûya of the house of the physician(s)". The question arises what function the *bīt asê* served. As shown by Joannès in the same article, it is normal for Late Babylonian ration lists to specify that food and medicinal substances were allocated to workers who were off sick, this condition normally being expressed by a form of *marāṣu* 'to be ill' (e.g. 1 *mašīḫu ša uṭṭati ana aklī ša marṣūti ardiya išši*(? gur$_{17}$) "one *mašīḫu* measure of grain for the bread of the sick ones (which) Ardiya *brought*," UCP 9/I 29, Joannès p. 75). CT 56, 618 fits this pattern if *bakûya ša bīt asê* means "Bakûya who is in the *bīt asê*", the *bīt asê* being a place where one went to obtain treatment and/or be taken into care.[52]

If the sick were sometimes accommodated in the "house"[53] of the healer, this may be the way to understand an Old Babylonian letter:

---

[48] For examples see *CAD* A/ii 345b.

[49] For an unusual case in which someone went to his *colleague* (*a-na* ɪʙ-*ri-šu*) for (medical?) inspection (*ana piqittišu*), was found to have a sick foot, and was bandaged before the king, see S. Sanati-Müller, "Texte aus dem Sînkāšid-Palast. Dritter Teil: Metalltexte", *Baghdader Mitteilungen* 21 (1990): 187: 15–18.

[50] Heeßel, *Diagnostik*, 369 fn. 53 and Joannès in *Médecine et médecins*, 143 fn. 34.

[51] CT 56, 618. See Joannès in *Médecine et médecins*, 84.

[52] Since dream interpreters also had a role in healing, the expression recalls the *bīt šā'ilāti* "house of the female dream interpreters" mentioned in Old Babylonian letters (AbB IV 145: 12 *bi-it ša-ḫi-la-tim*, VIII 78: 8′ é? *ša-ḫi-la-tim*).

[53] As recognized in Joannès's translation of *bīt asê* as "une structure appelée la 'maison des médecins'" (and in keeping with many other phrases which include *bītu* "house"), the phrase *bīt asê* does not necessarily imply that the *asû* lived on the premises, and could simply designate his workplace.

AbB XIII 66: 5–10 (Ibni-Marduk)

*aššum amtim ina–šamê–re-ša-*AM *ša abī atta / tušīrâšši-ma taddinašši / ana idiša ana bēltiša ša kanikkī ša arḫiš ēzibu / adi alākika ar-*DI*-i* 6 *ūmī irrūša išarū /* 2 *ūmī iṣne-ma ina bīt* ᵈ*na-bi-um–mu-ša-*[*li*]*m / ūšib*
Concerning the slave-girl Ina-šamê-rēšat whom you, my father, gave me by sending her: until your departure I *ar-di*?*-i* my sealed document, which I hastily drew up, concerning her rent for her mistress. For six days she had (regular) bowel movements, for two days she had loose stools and stayed in the house of Nabium-mušallim.

The context suggests that the slave-girl stayed in the house of Nabium-mušallim because of her stomach complaint, i.e. presumably to be cured of it. Healing may also be implied as the reason for a sojourn in other letters, but the interpretation is more dubious.[54]

It deserves mention that evidence for patients being removed to a place of cure has been sought in a group of Middle Babylonian letters from Nippur, mostly written in a short space of time (days or weeks)[55] by a healer named Šumu-libši.[56] Šumu-libši writes reports on the well-being of several, usually female, young patients,[57] afflicted with complaints which include fever (*ummu*), *abscess* (*išātu*),[58] coughing (*ganāḫu*, *su'ālu*), and *kīs libbi*. The addressee of the letters is Šumu-libši's 'lord', who, since communications with him are in writing and a messenger (*mār šipri*) is used, is probably located in a different building. Waschow

[54] E.g. AbB XI 36: 5–7 (Ištar-ēkallī to Kuk(k)uya) *ištu ana bīt nabium-mālik / ērubam šīrī matīma / ul iṭīb* "Since I entered the house of Nabium-mālik, I have never felt well (lit. 'my flesh has never been good')".

[55] H. Waschow, "Babylonische Briefe aus der Kassitenzeit," *Mitteilungen der Altorientalischen Gesellschaft* 10/I (1936): 25–40. English translation in S. Parpola, *Letters from Assyrian Scholars to the Kings Esarhaddon and Assurbanipal* II, Alter Orient und Altes Testament 5/2 (Verlag Butzon & Bercker Kevelaer, 1983), Appendix Q, 492–496.

[56] For this reading of the name (as opposed to Mukallim) see W. von Soden *apud* W.G. Lambert, "Ancestors, Authors, and Canonicity (JCS XI, 1–14): Additions and Corrections" *Journal of Cuneiform Studies* 11 (1957): 112 (and cf. Sassmannshausen, *Beiträge*, 73 fn. 1171). Šumu-libši's profession in not stated, but he is known to have been a functionary of the Gula temple (see Volk, *Orientalia* 68 (1999): 7 fn. 41).

[57] Ritter, *Studies Landsberger*, 317b "youngsters", 318b "children"; cf. Volk, *Orientalia* 68 (1999) 7–8 esp. fn. 43. There is also a lexical basis for this view: as argued by Landsberger and Roth, there is a word *na'r(t)u* meaning "youngster", and W. Farber, *Schlaf, Kindchen, Schlaf! Mesopotamische Baby-Beschwörungen und -Rituale*, Mesopotamian Civilizations 2 (Winona Lake, IN: Eisenbrauns, 1988), 55–56 (where refs. to Landsberger and Roth may be found) has persuasively suggested that this (rather than *nāru* 'singer', so Waschow and others) is the word attested in the Šumu-libši correspondence.

[58] See discussion by Stol in *Disease in Babylonia*, 21.

characterised Šumu-libši's place of work as a "eine Klinik", so that the letters offer a glimpse into nothing less than "den Betrieb eines babylonischen Krankenhauses".[59]

However, several features of the letters suggest that the patients were being treated in the building where they were normally housed. Šumu-libši himself seems not to live on the premises, for his instructions are: to learn in the evening what has happened in the day, to learn at dawn what has happened overnight, and to report to his lord accordingly (BE 17/1 33 = *LAS* II 495, r. 8′–12′). Indeed, one letter (BE 17/1 47 = *LAS* II 492) constitutes a report on a patient's condition overnight and at dawn, but Šumu-libši says he will despatch his messenger after he has learned more (*ṭēma alammad* [x]*x-bi-ir-ma* [*mār šip*]*riya uš*[*ēṣâ*]): apparently he wrote the letter immediately after arriving and speaking briefly to the patient's nocturnal carers, but before having had time to form a properly informed opinion.[60] Finally, several of Šumu-libši's letters open with the statement that the *na'rus* and *na'rtus* (see fn. 57) are well, then go on to discuss individual patients. In PBS 1/2 71 (= *LAS* II 493), where it is initially said that the *na'rus* and the lord's 'household' (*bītu*) are well, four reports out of six on individual patients are unfavourable. This suggests that the initial positive phrase should be understood as a general indication of the state of things, and not as a report directly on the patients. If Šumu-libši was in a position to comment generally on the state of things, we may suppose him to have seen more of his lord's affairs than just his patients. The impression we get, then, is that the *na'rus* are lodged in some sort of institution, perhaps (with Waschow) one connected to the temple, and that when some of them are ill Šumu-libši makes twice-daily visits, giving instructions for how they should be treated, observing progress, and reporting to their master – not just on the patients, but also on how the denizens of the institution are faring in general.

Thus the Nippur letters themselves are probably not evidence for patients being taken into care in a building other than their normal abode, but indications to this effect can be found in other sources.

---

59 Waschow, *MAOG* 10/I (1936): 25.

60 Further, it is said of two patients who have made a full recovery that *šumma bēlī išappara līṣânim-ma ana iḫzi līšibā* 'If my lord (so) writes, they may go out and attend instruction' (BE 17/1 31, *LAS* II p. 494, 9–10). Had they been removed to a special structure during illness, one might expect the note of dismissal to refer to their returning to their normal abode.

3. *Availability and Affordability*

Though the medical corpora and other sources amply attest to the existence of healers, it is far from clear who could resort to them, or how easily.[61] Food for thought is offered by I.L. Finkel, who cites an ethnographic parallel from the 1896 diary of a British army officer stationed in Kashmir and suggests that 'this state of affairs is probably a fair summary of what medicine had to offer the common man in ancient Mesopotamia': 'There is a man who has a book of fever cures which is said to be good, but as he wanders from village to village, he may be 50 miles off when required'.[62]

Sure enough, the issue of availability of practitioners surfaces in Mesopotamian sources. An Old Babylonian letter from Tell ed-Dēr contains a veritable cry from the heart:

> **IM 49233: 4–10** (al-A'dami, *Sumer* 23 (1967):[63] 157; Nidin-Ištar to Ikupiša)
>
> *ana nābi-ilišu asî / aštanapparam-ma / ulā illakam / šumma aḫī atta / ṭurdaššu-ma / simmam / līmur-ma*
>
> I keep on writing to the *asû* Nābi-ilišu, but he does not come. If you are my brother, dispatch him so that he will examine the sore and …

Below we will encounter another Old Babylonian letter (AbB VI 22) in which it is said that 'there is no haruspex in the village', causing the writer delay in obtaining divination. Healing and related professionals were not, therefore, always easy to come by.[64]

---

[61] The ancient sources themselves recognise that different social classes could aspire to different ritual practices. See the address to Šamaš published in A.L. Oppenheim, *The Interpretation of Dreams in the Ancient Near East. With a Translation of an Assyrian Dream-Book*, Transactions of the American Philosophical Society 46 (Philadelpia: American Philosophical Society, 1956), 301 and 340, which prescribes that the diviner bring cedar, the widow flour, the poor lady oil, the rich man a lamb. Note also J. Nougayrol "Aleuromancie babylonienne", *Or NS* 32 (1963): 381–386, who publishes a late Old Babylonian tablet of flour omens and observes that these were probably for use by the poor (who could not afford extispicy).

[62] I.L. Finkel, "Magic and Medicine at Meskene," *Nouvelles Assyriologiques Brèves et Utilitaires*, 1999/2, 28–30 n. 30.

[63] K. Al-A'dami, "A new Kudurru of Maroduk-nadin-ahhe: IM. 90585", *Sumer* 38 (1982): 121–133.

[64] In the Mari corpus, the king is asked by Itūr-asdu to despatch an *asû* because otherwise there will be no one available to cure anyone hit by a sling stone (ARM II 127). As observed by Durand, AEM I/1, 555, the author of the letter is getting ready for the siege of Naḫur, and foresees the need for specialist treatment of war wounds. The letter is, therefore, a special case, and does not prove that other types of medical treatment were unavailable in the town.

Besides the issue of availability, there was that of payment.[65] Indications from the professional corpora are limited to a small number of cases in which payment to the practitioner was incorporated into the ritual.[66] The *Codex Hammurapi* prescribes that different classes of citizen should pay different rates for the same treatment (§§ 215–223),[67] but the extent of the Codex's practical implementation is unclear, so the generalization that 'fees were graded according to the patient's ability to pay'[68] is problematic.[69] Indeed, the author of an Old Babylonian letter complains to her correspondent that she cannot afford the medical care she needs:[70]

AbB X 55: 15–17 (Ka-aya to Abâ and Bitî)

miqtum imqutam-[*m*]*a / ša ana a-si-im anaddinu / ul īšu*

miqtu has befallen me and I have nothing to give the *asû*.

Since hyperbolic complaints (hunger, nakedness, etc.) are standard in Old Babylonian letters, we need not believe the writer's declaration to be literally true. Nonetheless it proves that, at least sometimes, patients were expected to pay the *asû* directly,[71] and suggests that (as one might expect) this payment could, in principle, be problematic. Confirmation of this is forthcoming from another Old Babylonian letter:

AbB XI 53: 5–23 (Sîn-ašarēd to Sinātum)

awīlum ša aṭrudakkum / ul qātum aḫītum aḫī / ṭuppī ul tīde aḫī / ana asî(a[!].zu) *umma atta-ma /* [*a*]*na awīlim lā teggu /* [*a*]*nākum annikīam /*

---

[65] There may be a reference to the payment of dream interpreters in AbB VIII 115: 5′: kù.babbar *ša-i-lu-ti-šu-nu* (does the morpheme *-ūt-* indicate an abstract noun or the plural participle? The reading *ša ilūtišunu* "of their divinity" would give poor sense).

[66] Cf. M.J. Geller, "Comment et de quelle façon les praticiens gagnaient-ils leur vie ?", *Le Journal des Médecines Cunéiformes* 10 (2007): 35. Geller's interpretation of the incorporation of payment into rituals ("[c'est] une certaine politesse entre patient et thérapeute. [Il fallait] déguiser le paiement en cadeau, le paiement faisant ainsi partie du rituel de guérison") depends specifically on the interpretation of *qīštu* as "cadeau", and is open to doubt. For while "present" is indeed a well-known meaning of *qīštu*, it is equally clear that already in the Old Babylonian period it was a standard term for "fee, honorarium" (see esp. *CAD* Q 279b and *AHw* 924a on the *Codex Hammurapi* §§ 228: 62 and 234: 8).

[67] Cf. also the Ur-Namma lawcode, mentioned in fn. 37.

[68] Scurlock and Andersen, *Diagnoses*, 10.

[69] Robson, *Religion Compass* 2/4 (2008) 464.

[70] It is interesting that the *asû* should be mentioned in connection with *miqtu*, for the same connection is made in the *Diagnostic Handbook* XXXIII 53–55 (see Heeßel, *Diagnostik*, 356 and 361).

[71] This confirms the "best assumption" of Geller, *BSOAS* 69/3 (2006): 463.

[(...) libbaka] u[ṭ]āb / [i]na bīt tamkāri / [š]a talaqqi'am / anāku libbaka / uṭāb ana pīḫāt kaspim / ša tanaddinu / anāku azzaz / šumgurum u qabûm / ittika-ma / ana panīya / 2 šiqil kaspam uṣur / ana ṣibûtiya

The man whom I despatched to you is not a stranger – (he is) my brother! Did you take no notice of my letter? (He is) my brother! To the *asû* you (*shall* say) this: 'Do not be careless with the man!'. I will satisfy [you] here myself. What you take from the 'house of a merchant' (i.e. whatever money you borrow), I will satisfy you myself. I myself will bear the responsibility for the silver that you are to pay. Negotiation (lit. 'persuading and talking') (I leave) with you. Save two shekels for *what I may need*.

The situation is this: Sîn-ašarēd despatched a man to Sinātum, and the man fell ill. Sinātum duly informed Sîn-ašarēd, but Sîn-ašarēd was alarmed by the scanty medical care which Sinātum intended to give him. Accordingly he wrote this letter to tell Sinātum that no expense should be spared, he will be reimbursed, and the *asû* should be instructed to do all he can (lit. "not to be careless").[72] Thus the *asû* expected to be paid from private funds, and his fee cannot have been negligible, for Sîn-ašarēd imagines that Sinātum might have to borrow in order to pay it.

The considerations of availability and cost of professional treatment must have meant that professional care was not always one's first port of call. We find a possible reflection of this in the following Old Babylonian letter:

AbB XI 57: 10–22 (Lamassī to Nūr-kabta)

anum-ma aštaprakku / pitâk[a] [p]e[t]e-ma / 2 qa šamnam ina karpatim / šakin šūbilam / awīlum / kalbum iššuk-ma / urakkaš šamnam / šūbilam / mimma ana rigimti / ēkallika / itti tamkārī / tanassaḫu / anāku appal

Now I write to you: open your *opening* and send me two quarts of oil placed in a pot. A man: a dog bit (him) and I have to bandage (him). Send me the oil! Anything you have to draw from merchants because of a summons from your palace, I will pay you back myself.

The writer has to bandage a man bitten by a dog. Given that he (she?) does not even have oil for the purpose, even though in Old Babylonian times bandaging with oil seems to have been the cure of first resort for all manner of ailments,[73] one doubts that the writer is a professional healer.

[72] Another usage of *egû* "to be negligent" in connection with bodily care appears in A XII/60: 12 (unpublished letter from Old Babylonian Susa, cited *CAD* P 16a) *ana pagrika lā teggi ina šalimtim lūmurka* "Do not neglect yourself, I want to see you in good health!".

[73] Durand, AEM 1/I, no. 278. See also S. Dalley et al., *The Old Babylonian Tablets from Tell al-Rimah* (London: British School of Archeology in Iraq, 1976), no. 124, on

4. *Non-Medical Activities of Healers: Šamaš-muballiṭ*

The medical corpora suggest that literate healers were versed in an extensive body of knowledge, which must have required considerable training to master. *Prima facie*, this likens them to modern doctors, who spend a long time studying, and then devote themselves to healing full-time. However, it is still far from clear how "professional" Mesopotamian healers were. We are generally poorly informed about how much time they were expected to devote to healing and related tasks (such as the performance of private or temple rituals), what other sources of income (if any) they had, and whether it was normal for them to have other duties. The medical corpora do not help us further with these questions. On the other hand, letters are more informative.[74]

One individual whom we can put under the microscope is Šamaš-muballiṭ, known from a group of Old Babylonian letters in which he is the author of some (e.g. iii.23–25, iii.40–42, x.101), addressee of one (viii.158), and mentioned in others (e.g. iii.27, iii.49–50, viii.148).[75] Though his profession is not stated, the letters allows us to assemble a rudimentary impression of his activities.

In one case, a correspondent is instructed to ask Šamaš-muballiṭ about an abnormal calf:

AbB III 50: 21–24 (Bēlšunu to Addaya)

li'āti gimil-erṣetim ul imḫur / ana šamaš-muballiṭ qibi / u ṭēm būri ša pīšu ina kutallišu / šamaš-muballiṭ šāl

Gimil-erṣetim has not received the cows. Tell Šamaš-muballiṭ, and ask Šamaš-muballiṭ about the calf whose mouth is on its back.

---

bandaging a feverish boy and AbB XIV 43: 16–18 (request for oil in the wake of becoming ill). Was one function of the oil in such cases to keep the patient warm? (Cf. refs. in *RlA* "Salbung").

74 Given their connection to palace environments, where full-time employment of healers is *a priori* likely, Mari letters and Neo-Assyrian scholarly ones are exceptional and not necessarily representative of other situations.

75 The archive, which also includes contracts dating from Hammurapi year 38 to Samsuiluna year 30, was located in a North Babylonian town called Lagaba. See W. Leemans, *Legal and Administrative Documents of the Time of Hammurabi and Samsuiluna (Mainly from Lagaba)*, Studia ad tabulas cuneiformes collectas a F.M. Th. de Liagre Bohl pertinentia SLB I/3 (Leiden: Brill, 1960), 1–6 and AbB III, v.

What is sought from Šamaš-muballiṭ is probably an interpretation of the ominous significance of the abnormal birth.[76] Thus he was probably versed in the interpretation of terrestrial omens.[77]

In another letter, Šamaš-muballiṭ himself writes that he has pronounced a prayer for cattle,[78] and duly been remunerated:

AbB III 42: 9–12 (Šamaš-muballiṭ to Bēlšunu)

damiqti lâti / qabi'at / kīma šaddaqdi / qīštum ūṣi'am

The prayer for the cows has been spoken. Like last year, payment went out to me.

In a third letter, it is said that Šamaš-muballiṭ will write a report on a correspondent's health:

AbB III 27: 5–19 (Abum-waqar to Šū-amurrum)

[*ašš*]*um sili'ti*[*ka*] *ša libbaka* / [*imr*]*aṣu-ma ta*[*špu*]*ram adi ṭēm si*[*l*]*i'tika* / *marduk-nāṣir ištu maškan-šapir*[ki] / *išpuram anāk*[*u id*]*ûm īde-ma* / [*an*]*a šu*[*lm*]*ik*[*a*] *u*[*l*] *ašapparam* / [*kīm*]*a marduk-nāṣir* / [*išp*]*ura*[*m*] *xxx-šu* / [*ana šu*]*lmika aštapram* / [*šumk*]*a u zikirka* / [*ma*?*-ḫar*? *mar*]*duk u zababa* / [*xxx*]*x ki li* [*xxx*] / [*ana*] [*ša*]*maš-m*[*u*]*balliṭ* / [*ašp*]*u*[*r*]*am-ma maḫri'a*[*m*] / [*š*]*a illakam šulum zumr*[*ika*] / *išapparam*

[Ab]out [your] illness which you have become [anno]yed about, and about which you wrote to me, until Marduk-nāṣir sent me a report on your illness from Maškan-šapir, *would* I have known about it and not enquired about your health? As soon as Marduk-nāṣir wrote to me, ..., I am writing to enquire [after] your [he]alth. [*May they bless*] your name [*before* Mar]duk and Zababa ... I wrote [to Ša]maš-muballiṭ, and he will write back about [your] bodi[ly] well-being with the first (messenger) that comes.

If, as documented above, Šamaš-muballiṭ interpreted omens and was paid for reciting prayers, it is probably no coincidence that here he was chosen to deliver a report on a person's health (though it remains unclear whether he was supposed to perform a physical examination of Šū-Amurrum, or to produce his report from a distance, availing himself of

---

[76] Cf. Durand, AEM 1/I, 241 for a Mari letter reporting an anomalous birth to the king.

[77] E. Leichty, *The Omen Series Šumma Izbu*, Texts from Cuneiform Sources 4 (New York: J.J. Augustin, 1970), 7–8, who discusses the letter, suggests that Šamaš-muballiṭ was a *bārû*.

[78] *CAD* Q 31a doubts the translation of AbB III, regarding the passage as obscure and rendering it "the good condition(?) of the cattle has been declared(?)". However, *damiqti X qabû* is a standard phrase for intercession with deities on behalf of humans (*CAD* D 64b), and the translation of Frankena, AbB III, "Der Segen ist über die Kühe gesprochen" remains persuasive.

divination). Another possible connection between Šamaš-muballiṭ and healing is that in AbB III 41 he requests a delivery of *annuḫaru*-mineral, which is (among other uses) known to have been used in rituals.

Taken together, these sources strongly suggest that Šamaš-muballiṭ possessed skills falling in the divinatory-magical and (whether or not this should be considered a subset of the former type) diagnostic-medical spheres. What becomes interesting in the light of these inferred skills is that in other letters the magico-medical side to his activities is completely invisible (though in X 124 he deals with birds of the temple of Ištar of Lagaba). In III 25 he says he has no donkey skins (which seem to have been requested of him) and promises to despatch a carpenter. In III 40 he says he has sent corn, in III 49 he is said to have given somebody a plot of land (*bītu*), and in VIII 158 he seems to have a supply of straw. The involvement with corn, land and straw encourages, but does not prove, the hypothesis that he appears in an administrative list from Lagaba which records the assignation of ten harvesters to one Šamaš-muballiṭ.[79] In III 40 he also explains the necessity of finding pitch to caulk a boat, and he is mentioned as having a boat in VIII 148. He seems not to have led a "surgery only" existence, but to have been involved in the practical administration of farming, consistent with his issuing instructions for calves to be allowed to *roll about* (*lišgarriršunūti*) in X 101.

A single individual is not necessarily representative of a category, but Šamaš-muballiṭ at least shows that prosopographic research into the activities of Mesopotamian magico-medical cognoscenti will be rewarding, and that we should not expect to find them all working full time as healers or the like.

5. *The Role of Divination*

In principle, examining a sick patient and using diagnostic tablets to produce a prognosis might be viewed as equivalent to examining a sheep's liver and using extispicy tablets to produce a forecast of military success: in both cases the observation of signs leads to a prediction about the future. For this reason, some scholars term the entries on diagnostic tablets "medical omens",[80] though this usage is resisted by

[79] See Leemans, *Legal and Administrative Documents*, no. 177 lines 19–20.

[80] Cf. R. Biggs, "Medizin," *Reallexikon der Assyriologie* 7 (1987–1990): 624b, but see the comment in Heeßel, *Diagnostik*, 4–5.

those wishing to highlight the differences between the two activities as recognised by modern science.[81] Regardless of whether diagnostic tablets should or should not be regarded as divinatory literature (though from a Mesopotamian perspective they probably should), at least their relevance to healing is solidly documented and well known. By contrast, though it is clear that other forms of divination played a part in healing,[82] uncertainty surrounds the nature of their involvement.

One use which divination served in connection with healing was to produce prognoses and diagnoses,[83] but we are ill informed about the practicalities. In particular, it is not clear what relationship existed between diagnosis/prognosis as performed with diagnostic tablets, and other forms of divination. The medical corpora are not helpful in clarifying this issue. We must, therefore, look outside the corpora for sources which allow us to monitor the practical use of divination in connection with prognosis/diagnosis.

As confirmed by a query to Šamaš, at Esarhaddon's court extispicy was used for diagnosis, i.e. to determine which deity was responsible for an illness:[84]

SAA IV 190: 2–7

naqiya ummi aššur-aḫḫē-iddina šar māt aššur / ša inanna marṣatu-ma qāt(ē) iqbi-damiq / ina bīri iššakunši ina muḫḫi immer niqê alpē dib.meš (D(t)√*k'l*?) / *kī murṣu annâ marṣátu / ina šalimti ina pī ilūtika rabīti / šamaš bēlu rabû qabí kunú*

Naqiya, mother of Esarhaddon, king of Assyria, who is now ill, was diagnosed through extispicy as having the 'hand(s) of the god Iqbi-damiq',[85]

---

[81] E.g. Scurlock and Andersen, *Diagnoses*, xx: "The [prognostic/diagnostic handbook] is often denigrated or ignored on the grounds that it is a 'sorcerer's manual' containing nothing more than omens 'predicting the future of the patient'. However, the *āšipu* was not a sorcerer, and his diagnostic/prognostic handbook is not a collection of omens. Instead, the entries represent the distillation of millennia of first-hand observations".

[82] See fn. 22 above. For a case in which boils were provoked artificially to produce a diagnosis on the basis of their colour (BAM 578 i 8–10) see Stol in *Disease in Babylonia*, 23.

[83] See J. Nougayrol, "Présages médicaux de l'haruspicine babylonienne", *Semitica* 6 (1956): 1–14 and Heeßel, *Diagnostik*, 76–77, with additional refs.

[84] See Joannès in *Médecine et médecins*, 144–145, and note SAA X 315 (see Stol, *JEOL* 32 (1991–1992): 48).

[85] SAA IV 190 translates "on whom the 'hand' of god Iqbi-damiq was placed in extispicy" (cf. Joannès in *Médecine et médecins*, 145: "La 'main' d'une divinité a été placée dans l'extispicine sur la personne malade"). However, this interpretation is problematic, and it is more likely that *šakānu* in IV 190 refers to the placing of ominous signs in the exta, as in *šākin šīr dumqi ina têrtiya* "(Šamaš) who places favourable omens in my

> *it was (so) interpreted* through sacrificial sheep and oxen: is it reliably decreed and confirmed, by the command of your great divinity, Šamaš, great lord, that she suffers from this disease?[86]

As interpreted here, this query (which is itself divinatory) serves to confirm a diagnosis obtained through extispicy. This reminds us that the arbitrariness which in principle is inherent in extispicy could be reduced by taking omens repeatedly, until the sought outcome was confirmed.[87]

This query cannot, however, be presumed to be representative of all contemporary practice: the Neo-Assyrian court had a large number of scholars and practitioners available, so that multiple diagnoses could have been obtained easily; and scholars at the Neo-Assyrian court seem often to have been rivals in the quest for royal favour,[88] so it is not difficult to imagine different groups attempting to discredit each others' diagnoses in the king's eyes. Accordingly, additional sources need to be sought.

Some useful indications may be gleaned from the literary prayer of the Babylonian righteous sufferer, *Ludlul*. The first Tablet is devoted to ill luck and social estrangement. While this has physical/physiological repercussions in weeping, anxiety and nightmares, illness as such is not mentioned. The sufferer seeks help from the haruspex (*bārû*) and dream interpreter (*šā'ilu*):

> ***Ludlul* I 51–52** (Lambert, *BWL* 32)
>
> *dalḫā têrētuya nuppuḫ(ā) adanna*(ud.da.kam)[89]
> *itti bārî u šā'ili alaktī ul parsat*
>
> The omen organs are confused and inflamed on the appropriate day. My oracular decision is not rendered for the haruspex or dream interpreter.[90]

---

extispicy", *CAD* Š/1 120b (cf. Heeßel, *Diagnostik*, 77 n. 11). The point seems to be that the extispicy established 'hand of Iqbi-damiq' as a diagnosis, not that the 'hand of Iqbi-damiq' was placed on the patient during the extispicy.

[86] For a different interpretation see I. Starr, SAA IV, translating *kī* as 'if'.

[87] See Durand, AEM 1/I, 27 no. 403: omens taken twice, presumably in the hope of an improvement.

[88] See D. Brown, *Mesopotamian Planetary Astronomy-Astrology*, Cuneiform Monographs 18 (Leiden/Boston: Brill, 2000), 44–47 and 240–242.

[89] For ud.da.kam = *adannu* "the appropriate day in the year to perform a medical ritual" see Stol, *JEOL* 32 (1991–1992): 58.

[90] For the interpretation and translation of this line see Tz. Abusch, "*Alaktu* and *Halakhah*: Oracular Decision, Divine Revelation," *Harvard Theological Review* 80 (1987): 29–30. The passage is quoted by Nabonidus, see H.-P. Schaudig, *Die Inschriften Nabonids von Babylon und Kyros' des Großen*, Alter Orient und Altes Testament 256 (Münster: Ugarit Verlag, 2001), 493 fn. 704.

This choice of professionals is matched in an Old Babylonian letter in which a mother reassures her daughter that she will take action in respect of an ill-boding omen:

AbB VI 22: 4–29 and 42–44 (Huzalatum to Bēltani)

aššum ṭēmim ša tašpurīm / ezub lā šapāriki / ittī ilappatanni-ma / aššumiki ana bārîm / u šā'iltim a[ll]a[k] / uznāya ana mannim / ibašše'ā ana mārtiya / šanītim-ma kī'am tašpurīm / mimma ana pagriki / lā tana''idī pé-er-ke-tum / annīttan ša bēltiya-ma / lubārki ša labšāt(i) / šūbilīm-ma / taqrīwtam / liṣbatū / ana aya-tillatī / šumma tātamrīši / lā tarašššiši / ul ašpurakkim / umma anāku awīltum / šārassa šanât / adīni ana nērebtim / ul ēli-ma ṭēm / bārîm ul ašpurakkim / ina kaprim bārûm / ul ibašši / . . . / ziqtī šūbilīm-ma / [š]iqqam luškunakkim / liblūnikkim

About the matter concerning which you wrote to me 'Apart from your not writing, my sign portends ill for me,' for your sake I will go to the haruspex and the lady dream-interpreter. Whom else should I pay attention to? To my other daughter? *[91] Thus you (further) wrote to me: 'Do not fear at all for yourself'. Are these, then, the *obstacles* of my lady? Send me a garment of yours which you wear, so that an intercession can be made. Aya-tillatī, if you see her, do not *befriend* her – did I not write to you as follows 'The woman's hair(do) is strange'? So far I have not gone up to *nērebtu* (which is why) I did not send you the haruspex's oracular finding. There is no haruspex in the village. ... Send me *ziqtu*-fish so that I can prepare fish sauce for them to bring to you.

It is striking that, as in *Ludlul*, two different types of professional are to be consulted. This puts one in mind of the modern desire for a second opinion.

Returning to *Ludlul*, professionals are again mentioned early in Tablet II, after the situation described in Tablet I has lasted a full year:

***Ludlul* II 6–9** (Lambert, *BWL* 38)

bārû ina bīr(i) arkat(u) ul iprus
ina maššakka šā'ilu ul ušāpi dīnī

[91] The phrase *kī'am tašpurīm* "thus you wrote to me" is used to introduce and/or round off quotations. The AbB editor supposed that it was here used to round off a quotation stretching from "Apart from your not writing ..." to where the asterisk is placed in the translation, i.e. "... my other daughter". This, however, produces a rather perplexing situation in which a mother has a bad portent herself, yet goes to the diviner for her daughter's sake, and promises to look after her daughter. A better sense perhaps obtains if, as in the translation above, the quotation is made to finish earlier, after "... portends ill for me". *kī'am tašpurīm* must then be used to introduce a quotation, i.e. "Do not fear at all for yourself". So long as the sense of *pé-er-ke-tum* remains obscure here, it is difficult to decide how "Do not fear at all for yourself" fits into the thought train of the letter.

zaqīqu abāl-ma ul upatti uznī
āšipu ina kikiṭṭê kimiltī ul ipṭur

The haruspex could not *get to the root of the matter* through haruspication.[92] The dream interpreter could not elucidate my case with incense. I sought the favour of the *zaqīqu* dream god, but he did not *enlighten* me. The *āšipu* did not dissolve the (divine) anger against me with a ritual.

The services of the haruspex and dream interpreter have been retained, and in addition an *āšipu* has performed a ritual.

Later in Tablet II a long list of bodily ailments appears, and this time professionals are consulted specifically about illness:

Ludlul **II 108–111** (Lambert, *BWL* 44)

sakikkīya išḫuṭu āšipu
u têrētiya bārû ūtešši
ul ušāpi āšipu šikin murṣiya
u adanna sili'tiya bārû ul iddin

The *āšipu* recoiled from my symptoms, and the *bārû* was confused by my omens. The *āšipu* could not diagnose my illness, and the *bārû* could not predict the duration of my malady.[93]

The two professionals perform complementary activities. The *āšipu* observes bodily symptoms (*sakikkū*) and is supposed to provide a diagnosis (i.e. identify the deity responsible for the symptoms?), the *bārû* observes divinatory omens (*têrētu*) and is supposed to produce a forecast of duration.[94]

Duration being closely related to seriousness, one can compare an Old Babylonian letter from Tell Al-Rimah, where divination is used to gauge the seriousness of a disease:[95]

---

92 Possibly: "could not predict the future". See Tz. Abusch, *Harvard Theological Review* 80 (1987): 31.

93 The passage contains three plays on words: 1) illnesses are normally the object of *šaḫāṭu* "to tear away" (see *CAD* Š/I 94a), whereas (with *CAD* Š/I 87a) in line 108 the homophone *šaḫāṭu* "to fear" (by-form of *šaḫātu*) is used; 2) in line 109 a spurious similarity in roots is achieved between *ušāpi* (√*wp'*) and *āšipu* (√*wšp*) [thus now also Attinger, *La médecine mésopotamienne*, 76], cf. perhaps. Gilg. XI 25 *muššir* (√*wšr*, imperative *uššir* expected in Standard Babylonian) *mešrâm-ma* (√*šr'*) "abandon wealth" for the same effect; 3) similarly in line 111 *adannu* … *iddin* (√*ndn*). The normal verb used to set an *adannu* is *šakānu*, so the use of *nadānu* here is probably paronomastic.

94 Stol, *JEOL* 32 (1991–1992): 57.

95 The translation incorporates two changes to the original edition: *itarraṣ* can now be assigned to *AHw*'s *tarāṣu* II "in Ordnung sein". The suggestion that *ḫīṭu ul ibašši* (lit. "there is no fault/sin") means "there is no cause for worry" in contexts involving disease was advanced by E. Ritter, *Studies Landsberger*, 302a and followed by Scurlock and Andersen,

Dalley, *Rimah* 65: 4–19 (Aqbahamu to Iltani)

> *aššum šārti u sissiktim / ša ṣeḫrim ša tušābilim / têrtam ana muḫḫi šārtim / u sissiktim ēpuš-ma / têrētum šalmā / ṣeḫrum ša qāt ilim elišu / ibbaššû mādiš-ma / itarraṣ / mimma ˹ḫī˺ṭum ul ibašši / u ištēn ˹ṣeḫrum˺ annikīam / qāt ilim elišu ibbaši / mimma ḫīṭum elišu / ul ibbaši / ša qāt ilim elišu / ibaššû šū-ma / ˹ṣeḫrum˺ ittarraṣ*
>
> Concerning the hair and fringe of the youth which you sent me, I performed an extispicy (to obtain an omen) about the hair and fringe, and the omens are favourable. The youth upon whom the hand of god rests will be absolutely fine, it is not at all serious. The hand of god rested on another youth here, it was not at all serious. The youth upon whom the hand of god rests (at the moment), he too will be fine.

The situation as it may easily be reconstructed from the letter is that the writer was sent some personal items (hair and clothing) belonging to an ill youth and requested to use divination to predict the course of the illness, a function very similar to that performed by the haruspex in *Ludlul* II. Interestingly, the diagnosis ('hand of god'), which in *Ludlul* II is performed by the *āšipu*, seems to be taken for granted and not very important in the Rimah letter. This recalls the Akkadian Gula hymn, in which Gula, goddess of healing, proclaims *[a]sâku bārâku āšipāku* 'I am an *asû*, I am a *bārû* (haruspex), I am an *āšipu*' in that order (*bārû* before *āšipu*).[96]

Another interesting feature of the Rimah letter is that the writer supplements his divinatory report with information about a patient who previously suffered from the same (or a similar) illness, and enjoyed a favourable outcome. The intention is evidently to offer his correspondent hope and confidence by citing a positive precedent. In this case, we can see that divination and practical experience were used, at the writer's own initiative, in complementary fashion.

Diagnoses, 691 *ad* 155. Cf. also the Old Babylonian phrase *ḫiṭītu ul ibašši* outside medical contexts, e.g. ARM III 12: 10–15 *sutû 3 bīrī eqlim ina purattim elēnum t[er]qa šaknū-ma kayyāntam illakūni-ma ittiya innammarū u iturrū ḫiṭītum ul ibašši* "The Suteans are occupying three double-hours' worth of field alongside the Euphrates above Terqa. They regularly come, meet with me, and go back. There is no cause for concern" and AbB I 22: 15–16.

[96] W.G. Lambert, "The Gula Hymn of Bulluṭsa-rabi," *Orientalia* 36 (1967): 128: 183. A seal also published by Lambert ("A Cassite-period seal inscription", *Nouvelles Assyriologiques Brèves et Utilitaires*, 1988/4: 56) reads *asâ[t] / gula / še'āšši / ile''e / bulluṭ[a] / pīt pîša / ṣabta kišib ša[maš]-/muballi[ṭ]* "She is a physician, Gula! Seek her! She is able to heal! Grasp her utterance! Seal of Šamaš-muballiṭ." It is suggestive that resort to Gula's "utterance" should be recommended. Divination may be meant.

The role of divination in obtaining prognoses probably underlies a prayer in *Šurpu*, where it is 'Adad, lord of extispicy'[97] who banishes disease:

Šurpu IV 94

lizziz šamaš bēl dīni lipaṭṭir arnī lizziz adad bēl bīri likkiš murṣu

May Šamaš, lord of law, intervene and completely undo my fault. May Adad, lord of extispicy intervene and banish the disease.

As divine overseer of the placing of ominous signs in animal livers, Adad may have been thought to have a certain amount of discretion in determining the content of the messages in the exta. With him, then, rested the authority to promise a swift end to illness.

In addition to generating diagnoses and prognoses, divination was also used to investigate the appropriateness of undertaking medical treatment. Perhaps the best evidence for this is a *Tamitu* enquiry preserved on a single manuscript:

Tamitu no. 25: 1–9[98]

šamaš MIN *annanna mār annanna ša inanna muruṣ ašî lū pašittu / lū lubāṭī marṣu-ma aklī u* ⟨⟨ninda⟩⟩ *šikara* (kaš.sag) *muṭṭû urrī / u mūšī inamziqu idallipu-ma ilūtka rabīt(u)/ īde ina l[ibb]i* ⟨*ū*⟩*mu annî annanna mār annanna liṣrim likpid-ma / annanna asû [l]ē'û lište''e-ma / ina muḫḫišu lu*(-)[(x)]x *dullu mala īdû līpuš-ma* xxx / *asûtu* ḪAR x gig *u* níg.gu$_7$ (*ukultu*?) *ša zumrišu innassaḫa ud-d*[*a-par-ma*] / *iballuṭ ilūtka rabīt*(*u*) *īde k*[*ī'am*]

[*t*]*amīt epēš* [*asûti*]

Šamaš, ditto (= great lord whom I am asking, answer me with a reliable "Yes"!). So-and-so, son of so-and-so, who is now sick with the *ašû*-sickness, *pāšittu* or *lubāṭu*, and is consuming too little bread and beer, (who) moreover grieves sleeplessly by day and by night – (as) your great divinity knows. On this very day should so-and-so determine and resolve to seek out so-and-so, a capable physician, and should he ... *over him* (and?) perform all the treatments he knows ...? Will ... *asûtu* ..., (and) the sickness and *pain* in (lit. 'of') his body be expelled and dr[iven] out, [so that] he recovers? Your great divinity knows, e[tc.]

A [*t*]*amītu* about performing [*asûtu*].

[97] For this epithet of Adad see D. Schwemer, *Wettergottgestalten Mesopotamiens und Nordsyriens im Zeitalter der Keilschriftkulturen: Materialien und Studien nach den schriftlichen Quellen* (Wiesbaden: Harrassowitz Verlag, 2001), 683 and 706.

[98] W.G. Lambert, *Babylonian Oracle Questions*, Mesopotamian Civilizations 13 (Winona Lake, IN: Eisenbrauns, 2007), 130–131 no. 25. Our translation is based on Lambert's, but in several places (esp. line 7) we understand the passage differently).

The central concern of the enquiry is hemerological: whether or not the day on which the enquiry is performed is propitious for medical treatment.

Further evidence for divination in connection with therapy is forthcoming from Esarhaddon's court, where Šamaš is asked about the efficacy or appropriateness of a particular drug,[99] but its representativeness of other situations must again be questioned.

More generally, Esarhaddon's queries to Šamaš preserve traditional sapiential injunctions, including the following:

SAA IV 317: 5–7

šumma ana epēš asûti teppuš-ma asû ana marṣi qātīšu lā ubbal bārû qību lā išakkan nipḫu tasrirru

If you perform (an extispicy) about practicing *asûtu* (i.e. the craft of the *asû*), the *asû* shall not lay his hands on the patient, the *bārû* shall not make a prognosis. Deceitful omen.

The phrase "the *asû* shall not lay his hand on the patient, the *bārû* shall not make a prognosis" also appears once in the therapeutic corpus,[100] and is frequent in hemerologies. The implication is that omens were taken before performing medical treatment. This agrees with an address to Šamaš accompanying a ritual against *māmītu*:

AMT 71,1: 40–41[101]

[*ina balika*] *šā'ilu qība ana šarri ul išakkan* x [(xx)]
[*ina balika* … *ana*] *marṣi qāssu ul u*[*bbal* (x)]

[Without you], the dream interpreter cannot give the king an interpretation [(…)]
[Without you, the *āšipu*?/*asû*?] cannot treat (lit 'b[ring] his hand [to]') a patient.

Given the proximity to divination by the *šā'ilu*, it seems that divination (superintended by Šamaš) was necessary for medical treatment.[102]

This is implied also in an Old Babylonian letter:

---

[99] SAA IV 187: 7 *ina šaqê šamme annâ* "by giving (him) this drug to drink", cf. 185: 2′.

[100] AMT 51,2: 2–6 +52,9. See Stol, *JEOL* 32 (1991–1992): 56.

[101] Edited by E. Ebeling, "Ein neuassyrisches Beschwörungsritual gegen Bann und Tod", *Zeitschrift für Assyriologie* 51 (1955): 167–179.

[102] The restoration of the professional who performs the treatment is uncertain: *āšipu* and *asû* are both possible; cf. *KAR* 26: 24 (ed. W.R. Mayer, "Das Ritual *KAR* 26 mit dem Gebet 'Marduk 24'," *Orientalia* 68 (1999): 150) and 4R 32 ii.44, cited *CAD* B 123a.

Eidem and Laessøe, *Shemshara* 34: 11–20 (Sîn-išme'anni to Kuwari)

aḫūka rā'[i]mk[a] / u anāku r[ā]'im[ka] / šalm[ānu] u bīt[ka šalim] / u šēpš[arr]i amatka / imraṣ-ma têrtam / ēpu⌜š⌝-ma / qāt ištar ušēli / inanna ittūḫ / šalmat u ṣuḫārū / mārūka šalmū

Your brother who loves you and I who love you are well. And [your] house(hold) [is well]. However Šēpša[r]ri, your maid, fell ill, so I performed an oracular enquiry and warded off (lit. 'lifted the hand of')[103] Ištar. Now she has recovered and is well. Also the young men, your sons, are well.

Since the act of taking omens by performing oracular enquiries (*têrta epēšu*) is not otherwise known to have been therapeutic *per se*, the writer seems to have checked that it was appropriate to perform treatment before undertaking it.

A treaty of Aššur-nērārī V asserts that *hurāpu anni'u issu libbi pitqišu lā ... / ... ana marṣi šēlu'a* 'This spring lamb has not been brought out of its fold ... for (divination concerning) a sick man'.[104] The medical use of the lamb may be to serve in extispicy for diagnosis/prognosis, or in extispicy for therapy.

Sources outside the medical corpora thus suggest that, at least in some situations, divination had an absolutely central role in healing, and the *bārû qua* prognosticator could, on occasion, be considered even more important than the *āšipu qua* diagnostician.

6. *The Composition of Pharmaceutical Prescriptions*

Mesopotamian pharmaceutical prescriptions do not explain the logic behind their composition.[105] In origin, they must have drawn on a fund of popular herbal lore incorporating centuries of observations of the efficacy of particular remedies for particular afflictions. However, this fund of knowledge was probably expanded and systematised by professional healers.[106]

---

[103] On the transferred sense of *qāta šūlû* "to lift the hand" see AbB XIV 121: 12 with comment p. 206.

[104] SAA II 2: 10′–11′.

[105] See also the remarks of Geller, *JMC* 8 (2006): 3–4. For the suggestion that compilers of therapeutic recipes felt they had to include a well-known popular physiognomic tradition see Stol, *JEOL* 32 (1991–1992): 55.

[106] For an example of the written tradition incorporating an oral recipe see M. Stol, "An unusual prescription: oral tradition?", *Le Journal des Médecines Cunéiformes* 10 (2007): 1–3.

A reflection of this may be found in the statement of some prescriptions that they are *latku* ("tested"):[107] testing new drugs before administering them to important patients is known to have been a significant concern.[108] The statement that some prescriptions are 'tested' looks like an attempt to reassure users of medical tablets who might have been wary of following a prescription with which they were not familiar.[109]

Some recipes ("simples") prescribe a single ingredient, others several ingredients, sometimes in large numbers. In such cases the suspicion arises that there was an element of discretion on the part of the therapist,[110] but it is noteworthy that a Middle Babylonian letter written by a healer observes that *naṣmattašu kī ē[siḫušu] šammi ašî bat[iq] u bēlī īdi kī ištēn šammu ibbattaqu-ma lā išalli[m]* "When I as[signed] a poultice for him, no *ašû* herb was available and my lord knows that if (even) one plant is missing, he will not recover (LAS II 495: 12–15)." At present it is difficult to know how widely this sentiment was shared.

By the first millennium (if not earlier), curative substances had begun to be surrounded by speculative thought. This is invisible in the prescriptions themselves, but attested in learned commentaries which associate curative substances with body parts and gods.[111] Conceptual overlays of this sort seem not to have been the sole preserve of theoreticians, but to have been effected also by healers who dealt with plants on a practical basis. A "therapeutic vademecum" written by an apprentice *asû*[112] (BAM 1 iii.40-iv.25) and *Uruanna* III (KADP 22 r.iv.13–37) quote plant

[107] See refs. in *CAD* L 112b. On assurances of effectiveness see E. Leichty, "Guaranteed to Cure", in *A Scientific Humanist: Studies in Memory of Abraham Sachs*, eds. E. Leichty, M. de J. Ellis and P. Gerardi, Occasional Publications of the Samuel Noah Kramer Fund 9 (Philadelphia: Babylonian Section, University Museum, 1988), 261–264.

[108] SAA X 191, Finet, *AIPHOS* 14 (1954–1955): 135, cf. Gilg. XI 298.

[109] One can hardly, however, conversely deduce that a prescription which does not call itself *latku* had never been used before.

[110] On the basis of similar recipes including large numbers of substances, Abusch, *Mesopotamian Witchcraft*, 58–59 and "Lists of Therapeutic Plants: An Observation," in *Studies Leichty*, 1–3, argues that prescriptions could be built up from bare lists of substances, ritual or therapeutic instructions being added secondarily. This in turn suggests that not all items in long lists were necessarily supposed to be administered to the patient, but that the therapist could choose between them.

[111] See refs. in M. Stol, "Pflanzenkunde", *Reallexikon der Assyriologie* 10 (2003): 505b–506a.

[112] E. Ritter, *Studies Landsberger*, 303 bottom fn. 14 suggested that "since the *asû* is recorded as scribe in no other text, we must regard" ^{lú}a.zu as an error for ^{lú}a.ba. See however BAM 394 (cf. Attinger, "La médecine mésopotamienne", 18).

omens from *Šumma ālu* (cf. CT 39 pl. 9, 1′–10′), so we can see that information about plants' curative and ominous properties were learned and stored together.

In this welter of vagueness about the origin and composition of prescriptions, invocation of sources outside the medical corpora is salutary. One subject on which they can throw light is the grouping of curative substances in medical recipes.[113] To this end, we will compare a number of plant lists (administrative, lexical, etc.) from the first millennium:

A (Neo-Ass.)	**C (Neo-Ass.)**	**D (Neo-Ass.)**	**E (Late Bab.)**	**F' (Late Bab.)**
CTN III 140	KADP 36 iv.26–41	SAA VII 146: 1–13	UCP 9/II 27[114]	CT 55 376 obv.3′–9′
giš *šu-nu-⟨u?⟩*	giš.*ere-nu*	eren	giš.eren	šim.giš.eren
giš šur.mìn	giš.šur.min	šur.mìn	giš.šur.mìn	šim.*šur-men-ni*
giš *dap-ra-nu*	giš.*dap-ra-nu*	*dáp-ra-nu*	šim.gír	šim.gír
giš.ses	šim.bal	šim.gír	šim.sal	šim.sal
giš.man.du	šim.šal	šim.sal	gi.du$_{10}$.ga	šim gi.du$_{10}$.ga
giš.li	šim.man.DU	šim.^{d}maš	šim.mug	[šim.g]am.ma
gi du$_{10}$	gi du$_{10}$.ga	šim.*kur-di-nu*$^{?}$	šim man.DU	
	giš.gam.MA	*kur-ka-nu-u*	šim.gam.ma	**F" (Late Bab.)**
B (Neo-Ass.)	šim.ses	*bu-uṭ-na-nu*	šim.*bi-dur-ḫu*	CT 55 376 r.2$^{!}$′–9$^{!}$′
Pra.Voc.Assur 124–140	šim.MUG	*ḫa-šá-nu*	giš.šim.ses	
ì.meš	šim.buluh	šim.bal	šim.[...]	[ši]m.eren
ì.meš kù	illu hal	gi du$_{10}$.ga	šim.illu buluh$^{!}$	šim.*šur-men-ni*
ì.meš bur	illu li.tur	[šim].l[i$^{!}$ (x)]	*ab-la-a-ta*	šim.gír
ì.meš du$_{10}$.ga	numun šim.gig		šim.QU[115]	šim.šal
ì.meš bár.ga	ú.*kur-ka-nam*		še.gú[.gal]	šim gi.du$_{10}$.ga
ì.meš giš.eren	ú.še.li		šim.*la-ad-nu*	šim.man.DU
ì.meš giš.šur.mìn			šim.li	[š]im.gam.ma
ì.meš šim.gír			šim.*ia-a-ru-ut-tum*	[šim.*la*]*d*$^{?}$-*nu*
ì.meš *dap-ra-ni*			šim.gú.tur	

---

113 On traditional groupings of plants see J.V. Kinnier Wilson, "Notes on the Assyrian Pharmaceutical Series URUANNA: MAŠTAKAL", *Journal of Near Eastern Studies* 64/1 (2005): 45–52 and, by the same author, "On the Cryptogams in the lexical and related texts," *Le Journal des Médecines Cunéiformes* 6 (2005): 1–21.

114 UCP 9/II 27 = Joannès, *Médecine et médecins*, 76.

115 šim.*qu-⟨un-na-bu⟩* (with Joannès), or an unusual spelling of *isqūqu*$^{?}$.

ì.meš ^{d}maš
ì.meš *sad-ru*
ì.meš gu_4.meš
ì.meš udu.meš
ì.meš šah.meš
ì.meš
ur.mah.meš
ì.meš ku_6.meš
ì.meš
mušen.meš

The order in which plants are listed is not exactly the same across the sources, but neither is it fully random: certain plants appear in groups. The similarity between the two Neo-Assyrian sources B and D is striking:

B	*erēnu, šurmēnu, asu, daprānu,* *nikiptu*
D	*erēnu, šurmēnu, daprānu, asu, šimeššalû, nikiptu*

There is also a strong resemblance between the two Late Babylonian sources E and F" and the Neo-Assyrian source C:

E	*erēnu, šurmēnu, asu, šimeššalû, qanû ṭābu, ballukku,* ŠIM.MAN.DU, *ṣumlalû*
F"	*erēnu, šurmēnu, asu, šimeššalû, qanû ṭābu,* ŠIM.MAN.DU, *ṣumlalû*
C	*erēnu, šurmēnu, daprānu, ballukku, šimeššalû,* ŠIM.MAN.DU, *qanû ṭābu, ṣumlalû*

Though they subsequently diverge, in the sections shown above the first seven ingredients of F" figure among E and C's first eight, while E and C have the same first eight except for *asu* vs. *daprānu*. Interestingly, this portion in which the three sources resemble each other closes in each case with *ṣumlalû*.

Something on which most of the sources cited in this section agree is that, when they appear at all, *erēnu, šurmēnu, daprānu*, and *asu* belong closely together, with the first two in that order. This tendency can be observed elsewhere, e.g. BAM 1 iv.6–8: (*erēnu, šurmēnu, daprānu*), and even in Nuzi: *AASOR* 16 77 10 (*erēnu, šurmēnu, daprānu, asu*). Curiously, however, the tradition seems not to have been pan-Mesopotamian: it does not appear in the great Babylonian lexical series Urra-hubullu. In Uh III (MSL 5) *asu* and *nikiptu* appear together as in source D above (III 93–94), but *daprānu* (*duprānu*) only appears eight lines later (III 102, cf. also III 208). The sequence *erēnu* – *šurmēnu* is respected, but these two plants appear at a considerable remove from *asu* and *daprānu* (III 217–225).

It thus looks as if, when medical recipes enshrine the sequence *erēnu šurmēnu daprānu asu* (see e.g. *CAD* A/2 343), this is a special case. The ingredients were not chosen independently, ending up next to each other fortuitously, but rather they were selected as a group, in accordance with a wider Mesopotamian cultural tradition.[116] This tradition requires study and attention in its own right, and further cases of groupings need to be sought. When (if ever) the therapeutic corpus is available in electronic form, statistical studies of the ordering of ingredients should prove rewarding.

7. *Conclusions*

We hope to have drawn attention to an issue which has long lurked in the collective unconscious of medical Assyriology, without however being confronted directly: the history of Mesopotamian medicine cannot be written from the professional literature of the ancient healers alone. Fortunately, other sources of information are available (esp. letters), and as more of the medical corpora are edited, it should prove rewarding to work towards a tighter integration and complementation of professional and non-professional sources.

[116] Stol, *JEOL* 32 (1991–1992): 49 has observed that certain illnesses appear in groups (see also N. Wasserman, "Between Magic and Medicine – Apropos of an Old Babylonian Therapeutic Text against the *Kurārum* Disease" in *Disease in Babylonia*, 50–52 on sequences of diseases in OB incantations). Stol suggests that they represent an "exemplary list or all possible illnesses ... the main categories of disease as distinguished by the Babylonians". Were *erēnu, šurmēnu* and *asu* / *daprānu* sometimes regarded as the basic trio (/quartet) of curative substances?

CUNEIFORM TABLETS ON EYE DISEASES: BABYLONIAN SOURCES IN RELATION TO THE SERIES DIŠ NA IGI^{II}-*šú* GIG

Jeanette C. Fincke

The vast majority of cuneiform medical tablets concerned with eye diseases[1] known so far are of Assyrian origin. This situation is purely accidental and basically due to the immense number of cuneiform texts excavated at Nineveh during the late 19th and the early 20th centuries. According to the colophon of the second of three tablets of the series DIŠ NA IGI^{II}-*šú* GIG "If someone's eyes are diseased", King Ashurbanipal himself wrote down the cuneiform signs reproduced on the tablet, and later checked and collated the text: *bulṭi ištu muḫḫi adi ṣupri . . . azugallūt* ^{d}*ninurta u* ^{d}*gula mala bašmū ina ṭuppāni ašṭur asniq abrē-ma* "medical treatments from the skull to the (toe-)nail . . . the higher medical art of Ninurta and Gula, as many as there are, I wrote on clay tablets, checked and collated (them)".[2] Although this is no more than a respectful description for tablets that have been written "in the name of Ashurbanipal", as is the case for almost all tablets written for his royal library, we can in all certainty conclude that in general Ashurbanipal adopted a positive

[1] See. J.C. Fincke, *Augenleiden nach keilschriftlichen Quellen. Untersuchungen zur altorientalischen Medizin*, Würzburger Medizinhistorische Forschungen Band 70 (Würzburg: Königshausen & Neumann, 2000), (hereafter cited as Fincke, *Augenleiden*).

[2] H. Hunger, *Babylonische und assyrische Kolophone*, Alter Orient und Altes Testament 2 (Neukirchen-Vluyn: Verlag Butzon & Bercker Kevelaer, 1968), 103 no. 329: Ashurbanipal colophon type "q": "Palace of Ashurbanipal, king of the (entire) world, king of the country Assur, to whom Nabû and Tašmētu presented wide understanding, who owns a bright eye. The choice of scribal art, whose skill no one acquired among the kings, my predecessors, medical treatments from the skull to the (toe-)nail, excerpts that do not belong to the series, the elaborate instructions, the higher medical art of Ninurta and Gula, as many as are formed, I wrote on clay tablets, checked and collated them, and placed them firmly in my palace for reading and being read." This colophon is preserved for the most part on BAM 15 rev. iv 48′–52′.

attitude to the conservation of cuneiform tablets and written knowledge,[3] and that he had ordered his scholars to compile this and other series.

The Structure of the Series

The compilers of the series DIŠ NA IGI^{II}-*šú* GIG "If someone's eyes are diseased", which comprises three library tablets with four column each, collected all the available sources that deal with symptoms of eye diseases and compiled a more or less detailed description of the correct treatments. A list of ingredients together with brief instructions about how to produce the medication (an ointment, eye drops, eye powder, or the like) may be given, or the wording of an incantation with a short description of the appropriate ritual may appear. The data concerning the symptoms were organized into a logical sequence (see table 1):[4] the first three of the four columns of Tablet I are devoted to the symptom of blood seen in the eye, the so-called "red eye". This is followed by symptoms caused by real foreign bodies in the eye, and moving on to sties, secretions, hairs, conjunctival swelling, membrane disorders, and so on (Tablet I iv–II i). Dysfunction of lachrymal glands, resulting in too many or not enough tears (*keratoconjunctivitis sicca*) is followed by diseased eye lids (GIG.GIR, *k/gurāru ša kappi īnā-šu* seems to correspond to *chalazion*, a sort of big sty, which can grow as big as a hazelnut), and jaundice, or rather *icterus*, when the conjunctiva and skin turn yellow. The compiler then describes the treatment of the combined symptoms of "membranes and shadow", which were individually mentioned earlier and will be again later. A short sequence refers to bad eyesight, which is followed by the large section about treatments for "shadow" in the eyes, which stretches to one and a half columns of Tablet II.

Tablet III is devoted to various other symptoms. *Photopsia*, when flashing lights are seen without any obvious source of light,[5] is one of the main symptoms of the well-known disease ŠU-GIDIM.MA or *qāt eṭemmi* "hand of a ghost"[6] (Tablet III i). The second column of the third tablet

---

[3] See recently J.C. Fincke, "The Babylonian Texts of Nineveh. Report on the British Museum's *Ashurbanipal Library Project*," *Archiv für Orientforschung* 50 (2003/2004): 119–125.

[4] All the symptoms are dealt with in Fincke, *Augenleiden*.

[5] See Fincke, *Augenleiden*, 240–241.

[6] For the eye symptoms of this disease, see Fincke, *Augenleiden*, 213–215.

deals with *diplopia*, which is seeing double or multiple images, blindness and night/day blindness. The last two columns of the third tablet are not preserved.

Different Traditions in the Series

The sources the scholar or scholars used to compile this long series of three tablets came from different traditions. This can be seen, for instance, from the instructions in BAM VI 515, copied by Franz Köcher. In column ii, the verbal form *teqqi* "you daub" referring to the correct usage of the medication is written in different ways: The most common way is by using the logogram MAR (column ii lines 51, 53, and 55), but every now and then one can find the word written syllabically in Akkadian as *te-qí*[7] (column ii line 35), or even more precisely as *te-eq-qí*[8] (column ii line 42). Some instructions hint at the effectiveness of the treatment by predicting *iballuṭ* "he will be healed" written with the logogram TI[9] (column ii lines 51 and 52). This does not mean that other treatments are less effective; it simply reflects a particular local traditional formulation, although we cannot discover the origin of it because of the lack of other sources. On the basis of the series "If someone's eyes are diseased" it seems that whenever the effectiveness (*iballuṭ*) is stressed, the prescriptions use a logographical writing for the way the medication is to be applied (e. g. MAR "you daub", KEŠDA "you bind"); *te-qi* or *te-eq-qí* "you daub" is never followed by *iballuṭ* or similar expressions. Unless this is accidental it could reflect different traditions; alternatively the differences may be explained by the availability of space.

Different traditions behind the series can also be detected within the sequence of procedures for the so-called magical treatment. The incantation begins with a sort of headline, KA-INIM-MA "its wording is ...", and the incantation itself is introduced by ÉN, *šiptu*, "incantation". The ritual associated with the incantation is introduced with DÙ.DÙ.BI "its procedure is ...".[10] But different traditions can be distinguished by the way the end of the ritual is marked. In most cases there is no special

[7] See e. g. BAM VI 510 i 23′, BAM 513 ii 10′, BAM VI 514 i 2′, 4′, 23′, BAM VI 515 ii 13–16, 35, iii 49′, 51′, 52′, 53′, 55′, BAM VI 516 ii 26′.

[8] See e. g. BAM VI 515 i 52′, ii 42.

[9] See e. g. BAM VI 515 ii 27, 51, 53, 64, BAM VI 516 i 72′, ii 18′, 22′, 24′, 29′.

[10] See e. g. BAM VI 514 iv 1 +22–38.

expression at all, some texts write TI or TI-*uṭ* for *iballuṭ* "he will be healed",[11] and others use *in*$_6$-*eš* "he will recover".[12]

Babylonian Medical Texts on Eye Diseases

Only a few medical texts on eye diseases written during the second millennium B.C. have been published[13] so far, not enough to establish the origin of the different traditions behind the series. However, there are Babylonian medical texts on eye diseases from the first millennium B.C., which can be correlated with the Ninevite tablets. The following texts are available:

Museum number	Publication	Provenance
VAT 17406	BAM IV 382	Babylon[14]
BM 132097	Geller, AfO 35, 22–23	of unknown provenance

These are the only two Neo-Babylonian tablets dealing exclusively with eye diseases to have been published: the text from Babylon (BAM IV 382) contains prescriptions for ointments for eyes. The individual instructions begin with a list of ingredients and end with the condition for which the ointment is to be used: for example, *te-qít šá bir-rat* IGI "ointment for *birratu* of the eyes". Similar instructions can be found on the tablet of unknown provenance (BM 132097), and a Late Babylonian tablet from Uruk (SpTU II 50, see below) seems to have some parallels with that tablet.

---

11 See e. g. BAM VI 514 iv 1.

12 See e. g. BAM VI 514 iii 21′, iv 33, 38, BAM VI 516 iii 10.

13 One tablet from the Ur-III period gives the instruction to use an ointment for eyes, see HS 1357 (TMHC NF I/II no. 357), see also M. Civil, *Revue d'Assyriologie* 55 (1961): 94, and H. Waetzoldt, "Miscellanea neo-sumerica, V; Kollationen zu A. Pohl, Rechts- und Verwaltungsurkunden der III. Dynastie von Ur = TMH NF 1/2", *Oriens Antiquus* 15 (1976): 324. An Old-Babylonian tablet from Nippur that collects medication for different parts of the body is the oldest known prescription for an ointment for eyes (HS 1883 = BAM IV 393). The Akkadian medical texts from Boğazköy date to the mid second millennium B.C. (KUB 4; 37; KBo 8; see Laroche, CTH, no. 809, and Fincke, *Augenleiden*, 8 and note 47). One medical text on eye diseases has been excavated in Ugarit (Ugaritica V no. 19). Medical texts from the second millennium B.C. hardly use any logograms, but write syllabically, whereas the texts of the first millennium B.C. prefer to use logograms.

14 See O. Pedersén, *Archive und Bibliotheken in Babylon. Die Tontafeln der Grabung Robert Koldeweys 1899–1917*, Abhandlungen der Deutschen Orient-Gesellschaft 25

Museum number	Publication	Provenance
VAT 14531	LKU 60; BAM IV 410	Uruk
W. 22664	SpTU II 50	Uruk
(W. 22307/16	SpTU I 31	Uruk)

Of the three Late Babylonian medical tablets on eye diseases from Uruk, one is a commentary. BAM IV 410 is a small fragment of a medical text, but there is not enough text to reconstruct even one of the four prescriptions. The obverse is concerned with treatments for diseases of the ear, and the reverse with eye diseases. The tradition preserved in SpTU II 50, a tablet that deals exclusively with eye diseases, is somehow related to the Neo-Babylonian tablet of unknown provenance (BM 132097) for the two tablets share nearly identical prescriptions. SpTU I 31 is a commentary on the fifth tablet of the diagnostic series SA.GIG, which describes the symptoms of diseases of the eye and predicts the outcome of the disease (usually "he will be healed" or "he will die").

A few years ago, Irving Finkel[15] published medical texts from an archive dating to the Achaemenid period that most probably came from Sippar. Within the group of medical texts – nearly all of them are school-tablets – there is one dealing especially with eye diseases (no. 12), and another referring to eye diseases on the obverse (no. 22). The instructions given on tablet no. 12 of this group are similar to those of the Neo-Babylonian tablets and of the Late Babylonian SpTU II 50 insofar as it first gives a list of ingredients before describing how to prepare the medication and stating the disease for which it is appropriate (no. 12 left side 26: [*te-qí-tu*$_4$] *šá* IGI^{II}.MEŠ-*šú* ⌜GIG⌝ "[ointment] for diseased eyes"). Although only the right part of the tablet is preserved, text no. 22 seems to give the description of the symptom first, just as in the series "If someone's eyes are diseased". So far, none of the instructions given in these Late Babylonian texts have parallels in other medical texts.

Although the number of Neo- and Late Babylonian medical texts specifically devoted to eye diseases is very small, one should keep in mind that treatments for eye diseases were also included in medical compendia dealing with other parts of the body. However, recently two more

(Berlin: Harrassowitz Verlag, 2005), 265: N15, 274 (findspot: 'Ischin-Aswad, M 27, Grube 31').

15 I.L. Finkel, "On Late Babylonian Medical Training," in *Wisdom, Gods and Literature. Studies in Assyriology in Honour of W.G. Lambert*, eds. A.R. George and I.L. Finkel, (Winona Lake, IN: Eisenbrauns, 2000), 137–223.

texts on eye diseases have been identified within the Babylon Collection of the British Museum:[16] the first of these tablets, BM 54641+54826, could well have been excavated at Borsippa.[17] The other one, BM 40737, is a fragment, possibly of a school-tablet – of unknown provenance. Together with the tablets published by Finkel we now have two more Neo-Babylonian and two more Late Babylonian texts concerned with eye diseases. These are the following:

New Neo-Babylonian Medical Tablets on Eye Diseases:

Museum Number	Publication	Provenance
BM 54641+54826	below	of unknown provenance, possibly Borsippa
BM 40737	below	of unknown provenance

New Late Babylonian Medical Tablets on Eye Diseases:

Museum number	Publication	Origin
BM 42610+43481	Finkel, FS Lambert, no. 12	Sippar
BM 42638+43262+43811 (obv.: eye diseases)	Finkel, FS Lambert, no. 22A[18]	Sippar
BM 43608 (+) F 239 (obv.: eye diseases)	Finkel, FS Lambert, no. 22B	Sippar

BM 54641+54826

BM 54641+ is the lower part of a one-column tablet on eye diseases measuring 7.23 cm by 8.2 cm. The thickest part of the broken tablet is 2.85 cm, but this would not have been the thickest part of the whole tablet, which can be supposed to have been 17 cm high. The surface of the upper part of the obverse is very badly damaged, but the reverse is

[16] Thanks are due to the Trustees of the British Museum for their permission to publish both tablets as well as the photos. I would like to thank Irving L. Finkel for reading the tablets with me. The transliteration and understanding of these very difficult to read tablets has been improved considerably during my discussions with him.

[17] So according to the expertise of Irving L. Finkel.

[18] Both fragments are copies of the same text and will accordingly be counted as one.

well preserved. This tablet[19] has been known to the wider Assyriological public since JoAnn Scurlock cited passages from it in "*Diagnoses in Assyrian and Babylonian Medicine*",[20] but there has been no edition of the entire text.

The format of the tablet begins with a description of the symptom followed by a list of ingredients and a short description of how the medication needs to be prepared and applied. One prescription, for example, reads as follows: "[If someone's eyes] are full of flesh and blood: myrrh, ammi, Ú.UD, (animal) f[at, *kanaktu*-plant, "spur of a bat"-drug] 4'[(and) cress] you knead [with] oil; (with this) oil [you daub his] eye[s]" (obv. 3′–4′). This is the standard format for prescriptions in medical cuneiform texts, and an identical prescription can be found in another medical text, written in exactly the same way with logograms (BAM I 22, a Neo-Assyrian text from Aššur). Other prescriptions in BM 54641+ can also be found in BAM II 159 (a late Middle Assyrian tablet from Aššur that collects prescriptions for symptoms on various parts of the body), in the first tablet of the series "If someone's eyes are diseased" from Nineveh in Neo-Assyrian script, and in the Late Babylonian text from Uruk SpTU I 50. A more detailed analysis of parallels between the prescriptions of BM 54641+ and other texts can be taken from a full transliteration and translation of this text:

[19] Some years ago Nils P. Heeßel kindly directed me to this tablet.

[20] JA. Scurlock and B.R. Andersen, *Diagnoses in Assyrian and Babylonian Medicine. Ancient Sources, Translations, and Modern Medical Analyses.* (Urbana/Chicago: University of Illinois Press, 2005).

obv.

1′ (traces)

2′ [_ _ _ _] ⸢U$_5$⸣.GAR.IB.MUŠEN *ina* ÚŠ GIŠ.ERI[N ḪI.Ḫ]I ZA.NA.DÙ-*uš* [*ina* A.MEŠ SÚD MAR]

3′ [DIŠ NA IGI^{II}-*šú*] ⸢UZU *u* ÚŠ⸣ S[I].⸢A⸣.MEŠ ŠIM.⸢SES⸣ ⸢Ú⸣.KUR.RA Ú.UD ⸢Ì⸣.[UDU ŠIM.GIG U$_5$.GAR.IB.MUŠEN]

4′ [*saḫ-lé-e ina*] ⸢Ì SILA$_{11}$⸣-*aš* Ì IGI^{I}[^{I}]- [*šú* MAR]

5′ [DIŠ NA IG]I^{II}-*šú* ÚŠ ⸢SI.A⸣.[MEŠ ⟨Ú⟩].UD [_ _ _ _ _ _ (_)Ḫ]I.[ḪI

6′ [DIŠ NA IGI^{II}-*šú* Ú]Š SI.A.MEŠ-*ma* _[_ _ _ _ _ _ _ _ _ _ _ (_ _)-E]N NA[M] MA$^?$/KU$^?$ ⸢Ú⸣.[_ _ (_)]

7′ [_ _ _ _] *ina* GEŠTIN ⸢SILA$_{11}$⸣-*a*[*š* _]_ _[_ _ _ (_) IGI^{II}-*šú*] LAL-[*id*]

8′ ⸢DIŠ NA IGI⸣[^{II}-*šú* ÚŠ] SI.A.MEŠ *ur-ri u* GE$_6$ *la* ⸢*i*⸣-[*ṣ*]*a-lal*-⸢*ma la ina-ṭal é*$^?$⸣-*kil* IGI^{II}-⸢*šú*⸣[21] [_ _]

9′ ŠÀ I[GI^{II}-*šú*] SA$_5$.MEŠ IGI^{II}-*šú* DUL-*ma* GAZI.⸢SAR *tur*⸣-*ár* ⸢KI Ì LÁL$^?$⸣ *i*[*na* G]A ⸢MUNUS.Ú⸣.[ZÚ]G

10′ SILA$_{11}$-*aš* LA[L *m*]*u*-⸢*kil* GABA⸣-*šú-ma* TIN-*šú* [N]A$_4$.⸢*as-ḫur ina* Ì.NUN SÚD IGI^{II}-*šú* MAR SUḪUŠ⸣ Ú.⸢*ra-pa*$^?$-*di*$^?$⸣

11′ ⸢*ina* GÌR⸣ Z[AB]AR ⸢KUD⸣ SÍK.Ḫ[É.ME.D]A SÍK.BABBAR NU.NU NIGIN-*mi tara-kas* SAG.KI^{II}-*šú* ⸢*ki*⸣-*lat*-⸢*tan*⸣ [LÁL]

12′ LÁ[L].⸢BI⸣ _[_ _ _]_-[*i*]*m*[22] ḪÁD.DU-*ma* IGI^{II}-*šú* [*t*]*e-e*[*q-qí*]

13′ DIŠ NA [IGI^{II} KI.MIN _]_ ⸢_⸣ *saḫ-lé-e ina* KAŠ ŠEG$_6$.GÁ SILA$_{11}$-*aš* M[AR]

14′ DIŠ N[A IGI^{II}-*šú* ÚŠ *šu-u*]*n-n*[*u-ʾa* NUMUN NÍG.GÁ]N.GÁN.SAR$^!$(DI) LÀL.KUR.⸢RA SAḪAR⸣ KÙ.GI 1-*niš* ḪI.ḪI S[ÚD MAR]

15′ [DIŠ NA] I[GI^{II}]-⸢*šú*⸣ [Ú]Š *iṭ-ri-ma* GUB-*iz* Ì.UDU ⸢Ì.NUN *ina* MUN NÁ⸣-[*a*]*l* ⸢ḪÁD.DU *ina* Ì⸣ S[ÚD MAR]

16′ [DIŠ NA] IGI^{II}-*šú šik*-⸢*na šá* ÚŠ⸣ *š*[*ak-n*]*a* ⸢Ú.UD$^?$⸣ ⸢U$_5$$^?$⸣.[GAR.IB.MUŠE]N ⸢MUN⸣.E[ME.SAL.LIM]

17′ [Ú].⸢KUR.RA Ú⸣.[KUR.KUR ŠIM].⸢GÚR.GÚR GAZI.SAR⸣ [_ _ _] ⸢_⸣ 8 Ú.ḪI.A Š[EŠ$^?$.MEŠ SÚD]

18′ *ina* ⸢ZÉ⸣ UDU.⸢NÍTA⸣ [ḪI.ḪI ZA.N]A ⸢DÙ-*uš*⸣ BE-*ma* EN.TE.[NA *ina*] ⸢A⸣.[M]EŠ BE-⸢*ma*⸣ AMA$^!$.MEŠ *ina* A ⸢GAZI⸣.SAR *ta-s*[*a-pan* MAR]

---

[21] The expression *ekil īnē-šu* "the dark (part) of his eyes" is unique, but could be compared with *namra īni* 'the light (part) of the eye' in AMT 59, 2 line 2′. This symptom is omitted in the first tablet of the series 'If someone's eyes are diseased', BAM VI 510 i 31′–32′ // BAM VI 514 i 38′–39′.

[22] BAM VI 514 i 42′ has: ⸢KEŠDA⸣.BI ⸢LUL GISSU⸣ ḪÁD.DU-*ma* "his bandage ... (in) shadow you let dry, and ..."

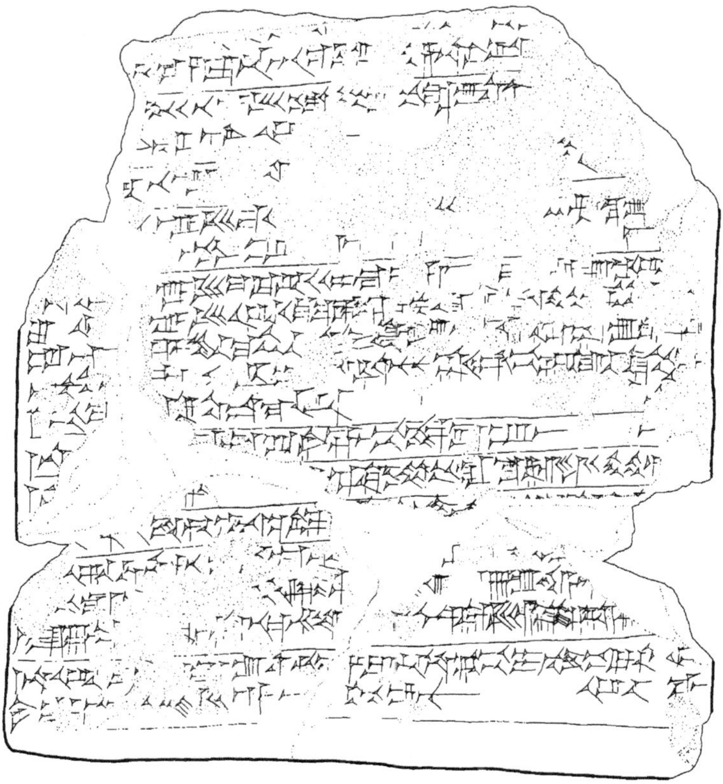

Figure 1: BM 54641+
(See corresponding figure 4; page 102)

19′ DIŠ NA IGI^{II}-*šú* ⌜*i*⌝-[*bar-ru*]-⌜*ra*⌝ Ú.UD ⌜U$_5$⌝.GAR.IB.MUŠEN NA$_4$.*ga-bi-i* MUN.EME.SAL.LIM

20′ Ì.⌜UDU⌝ Š[IM.GI]G 1-*niš* SÚD *ina* [Ì].*gu-un-nu* IGI^{II}-*šú* MAR

rev.

1 DIŠ KI.MIN ŠIM.ŠEŠ Ú.UD U$_5$.GAR.IB.MUŠEN *ina* Ì.NUN.NA SÚD MAR

2 DIŠ KI.MIN 1 GÍN U$_5$.GAR.IB.MUŠEN 1/2 GÍN Ú.UD 14 ŠE MUN.EME.SAL.LIM IGI^{II}-*šú te-eq-qí*
3 *te-qí-ti šá ḫa-am⟨-mu⟩-r[a-b]i* *la-ti-iq-ti*

4 [DIŠ NA] ⸢IGI⸣^{II}-*šú i-bar-ru-r[a ù* É]R ⸢*ú-kal*⸣*-la* Ú.UD LÀL KUR.RA *ina* Ì.⸢SAG⸣ S[ÚD MAR]

5 ⸢DIŠ NA IGI^{II}-*šú* ÉR SI.A⸣.[MEŠ]_ *ina* KAŠ SILA$_{11}$-*aš* LÁ[L][23]

6 DIŠ NA IGI^{II}-*šú* ÉR *im-l[a*$^?$*]-*⸢*a* __ __ __ __ __ __ __ __⸣ [
7 15 ŠE Ú.UD *ina* Ì.UDU ⸢*rib*⸣*-qí* SÚD [MAR]

8 DIŠ NA IGI^{II}-*šú lu* ÉR (over erasure) ⸢*lu* ZÁḪ⸣ ŠUB.ŠUB.A[24] *saḫ-lé-e ina* KAŠ.Ú.SA SILA$_{11}$-*aš* [LAL]

9 [DIŠ N]A IGI^{II}-*šú* LÙ.LÙ-⸢*ḫa*⸣ LÀL Ì.NUN.NA Ì.⸢SAG⸣ 1-*niš* ḪI.ḪI *ina* GE$_6$ IGI^{II}-*šú* ⸢SI.A⸣

10 [DIŠ NA IG]I^{II}-*šú ri-šu-*⸢*ta*$_5$⸣ SI.A.MEŠ *kam-mu šá* LÚ.AŠGAB *ina* ⸢LÀL⸣.ḪÁD MAR

11 [DIŠ NA IGI^{I}]^{I}-⸢*šú i*⸣*-pi-*⸢*ta*$_5$⸣ *bir-ra-ta*$_5$ *u gu-qa-na ú-kal-la* Ú.UD NAGA.SI ⸢__ __⸣

12 [T]I-*qé* UGU-*ḫi šá* GÌR.PAD.DU UDU NÍTA ḪI.⸢ḪI⸣ IGI^{II}-*šú* MAR-*ma ina-*⸢*eš*⸣

13 [DIŠ NA IGI^{II}-*šú bir-r]a-ta*$_5$ *a-šá-a* SA$_5$.⸢MEŠ⸣ 1 GÍN Ú.UD 1/2 GÍN NA$_4$.*ga-bi-i* IGI.4.G[ÁL.L]A
14 [IGI.X.G]ÁL.L[A M]U[N.E]ME.SAL.LIM 1 GÍN GAZI.SAR 1 GÍN Ú.KUR.⸢RA⸣
15 [_]_ 1 GÍ[N] ⸢Ú⸣.KUR.KUR 1 GÍN ⸢ŠIM⸣.GIG 1 GÍN Ú.MAŠ.TAB.⸢BA⸣
16 [G]ÍN Ú.⸢ḪAR⸣.ḪAR 1 GÍN Ú.NAGA.SI 1 GÍN ⸢Ú⸣.*t[a-ḫa*$^?$*-z]u*$^?$
17 [ ]⸢Ú$^?$⸣.[IGI]-NIŠ Ú.SI.SÁ 16 Ú.ḪI.⸢A⸣ [

18 [ ] (traces) [
(rest of reverse is missing)

[23] This prescription could probably be identified with BAM II 159 v 1–2: [DIŠ NA IGI^{II}-*šú*_]_-⸢RE ŠU⸣ *saḫ-lé-e* ⸢Ú⸣.[__ __] ^{2}*ina* KAŠ SILA$_{11}$-*aš* [LAL] "[If someone's eyes are .]...: cress (and) [...]-plant you kneed in beer (and) [bandage (with this)]".

[24] Scurlock, *Diagnoses*, 192 § 9.43 interprets the description of the symptoms in BAM II 159 v 3, which is parallel to this one, differently; she reads: DIŠ NA IGI^{II}-*šú lu* ÉR *lu-ḫa-a* ŠUB.MEŠ "If a person's eyes continually shed dirty tears ..."

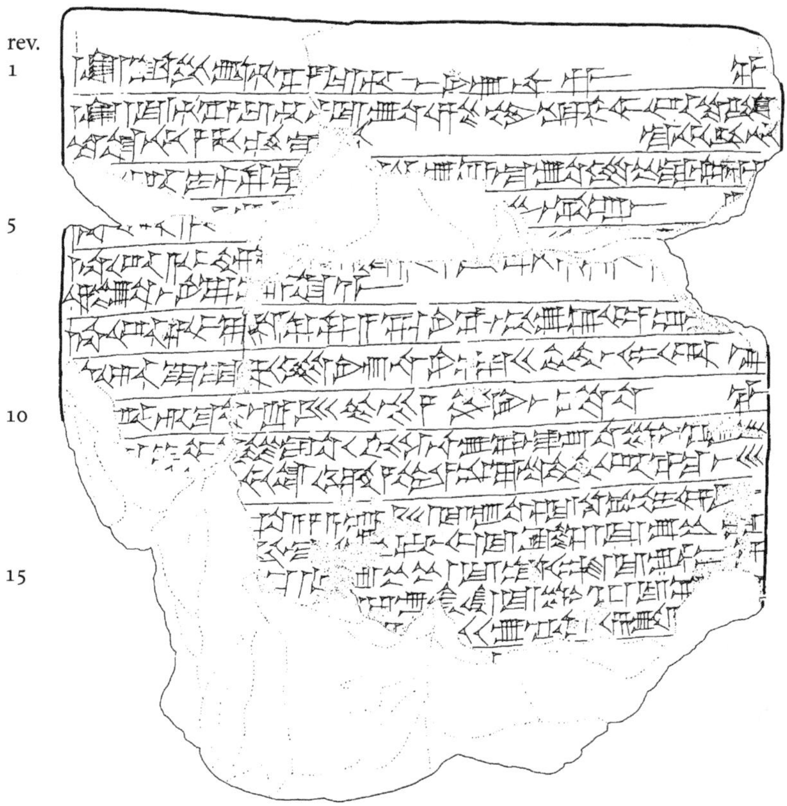

Figure 2: BM 54641+
(See corresponding figure 5; page 103)

Translation:

obv.

1′ (traces)

2′ […] "spur of a bat"-drug [you mi]x with cedar-blood, produce a doll, [grind (it) with water and daub (his eyes)].

3′ [If someone's eyes] are full of flesh and blood: myrrh, ammi, Ú.UD, (animal) f[at, *kanaktu*-plant, "spur of a bat"-drug]

4′ [(and) cress] you knead [with] oil; (with this) oil [you daub his] eye[s].

5′ [If someone's ey]es are full of blood: ⟨Ú⟩.UD, [… … you m]ix [up …].

6′ [If someone's eyes] are full of blood and .[...] .... .[...]
7′ [...] you knead with wine, [...]; (this mixture) you apply (in a bandage to) [his eyes].

8′ If someone's eye[s] are full of [blood], day and night he cannot sleep, and he cannot see; the dark (part) of his eyes [...],
9′ the inside of [his] e[yes] is (completely) red and his eyes are covered: you parch mustard and together with oil (and) honey i[n mi]lk of a ritually unclean woman;
10′ you knead (this) and apply (in a bandage). (It is the demon) 'who holds back his breast'! (For) his cure you grind *asḫur*-mineral in butter (and) daub his eyes; root of the *rapādu*-plant,
11′ you cut with a b[ron]ze knife; you spin white and red wool, surround (and) bind (this); both temples [you bandage (with this)];
12′ his bandage ... you dry up, and his eyes [y]ou d[aub].

13′ If someone's [eyes are ditto:] you cook [..]. (and) cress in beer, knead (it) and da[ub (his eyes)].

14′ If someo[ne's eyes are bl]ock[ed with blood: seeds of *sisymbrium off*]*icinale*, honey and gold-dust you mix up all together, gr[ind (this), and daub (his eyes)].

15′ [If bl]ood penetrates [someone]'s e[yes] and it stays: you lay (animal) fat (and) butter in salt, dry (this), gri[nd (this)] with oil, [(and) daub (his eyes)].

16′ [If someone's] eyes have a layer of blood: Ú.UD$^{?}$, "sp[ur of a ba]t"-drug, e[*mesallu*]-salt,
17′ Ammi, [*atā'išu*], *kukuru*, mustard, [...].; [you grind] (these) 8 bi[tter (?)] ingrediences
18′ [mix] (them) with bile from a male sheep, (and) produce a [do]ll; if it is cold, ... [you daub his] eyes.

19′ If someone's eyes *ibarrurā*: Ú.UD, "spur of a bat"-drug, alum, *emesallu*-salt,
20′ (animal) fat (and) *kanaktu* you grind all together (and) with [oil] of average quality you daub (this) on his eyes.

---

rev.

1 If ditto: myrrh, Ú.UD (and) "spur of a bat"-drug you grind with butter and daub (his eyes).

---

2 If ditto: (with) 1 shekel of "spur of a bat"-drug, 1/2 shekel of Ú.UD, 15 grains *emesallu*-salt you daub his eyes.
3 Tested ointment of Ḫammurapi.

---

4 [If someone's] eyes *ibarrurā* [and] hold [te]ars: Ú.UD (and) honey you gri[nd] in first class oil [(and) daub (his eyes)].

---

5 If someone's eyes are full of tears: you knead [... (and) ..]. in beer (and) you band[age (with this)].

---

6 If someone's eyes fill up with tears: ...
7 15 grains of Ú.UD you grind in boiled down (animal) fat [(and) daub (his eyes)].

---

8 If someone's eyes are thrown either into tears or 'into lost': you knead cress in *billatu*-beer [and apply (in a bandage to his eyes)].

---

9 [If some]one's eyes are constantly blurred: you mix together honey, butter (and) first class oil and fill (this) onto the pupil of his eyes.

---

10 [If someone's ey]es are full of redness: you dry *kammu* of the leatherworker (mixed) in(to) white honey and daub (his eyes).

---

11 [If someone's eyes] "hold clouding over", *birratu* or *qūqānu*: Ú.UD, salicornia, ...,
12 [...] you [ta]ke, on top of a bone of a male sheep you mix (it), (then) smear on his eyes, and he will recover.

---

13 [If someone's eyes] are troubled (*ešû*) because of [*birr*]*atu* (and) are red: 1 shekel of Ú.UD, 1/2 shekel of alum, 1/4 [shek]el
14 [of ..., ...], 1/[x] (shekel) of *emesallu*-salt, 1 shekel of mustard, 1 shekel of ammi,
15 [... ..]. 1 shekel of *atā'išu*-drug, 1 shekel of *kanaktu*-drug, 1 shekel of *māšu*-plant,
16 [... sh]ekel of thyme, 1 shekel of *salicornia*, 1 shekel of *t*[*aḫaz*]*u*-drug,
17 [...,] *imḫur-ešrā*, *šurdunû*-plant; (these) 16 drugs [...]

---

18 [ ] (traces) [
(rest of reverse is missing)

Commentary:

Because there are parallel entries for most of the given prescriptions, details in earlier commentaries will not be repeated. Some comments have already been given in footnotes, and others will be included in the following survey on the structure of this text.

Structure of BM 54641 + 54826 (See Table 2):

The first symptom described on the obverse of BM 54641+ could possibly be the same as on BAM I 22 obv. 4′–8′, which is restored from Tablet II of the series "If someone's eyes are diseased" (BAM VI 515 i 22′–24′): DIŠ NA IGI^{II}-*šú* UZU DU-*ka* SI.[A-*ma u* DU-*a*]*k ana* TI-*šú* (5′) *saḫ-lé-e* Ú.KUR.KUR ŠI[M ŠE]Š Ì.UDU ŠIM.GIG (6′) Ú.UD U$_5$.GAR.IB.MUŠEN MU[N.EME.S]AL.LIM 1-*niš* SÚD (7′) *ina* ÚŠ ERIN *lu ina* Ì ER[IN] ḪI.ḪI ZA.NA DÙ-*uš* (8′) *ina* A.MEŠ SÚD MAR "If someone's eyes are fu[ll of] 'growing / moving' flesh [and it move]s, to cure him: cress, *atā'išu*-plant, myrrh, *kanaktu*-tree resin, Ú.UD, "spur of a bat"-drug, [*emes*]*allum*-salt, grind (them) together and mix (them) with cedar resin ('blood') or cedar oil, produce a doll, grind (this) with water, daub (his eyes)". What remains of the instructions in BM 54641+ obv. 1′ is similar to that prescription, which suggests that the first sequence of the broken tablet deals with eyes full of "moving" or "growing" flesh. This fits well with the next symptom described as eyes that "are full of flesh and blood". Blood is the subject of the following seven prescriptions (obv. 5′–18′). The first three refer to eyes full of blood in combination with other symptoms, and the others seem to deal with real blood flowing from injured eyes.

The next four prescriptions (obv. 19′–rev. 4) deal with the symptom called *barāru*, which refers either to a general irritation of the eyes that makes them flicker, or to a sort of dimness of the eyesight.[25] The symptom of *barāru* is combined with tears in reverse line 4, which precedes a section dealing with tears. Reverse 8 has the symptom of eyes that are thrown either into tears or into ZÁḪ, an obscure expression literally meaning "in lost".[26] Except for reverse line 10, which deals with the redness of the eyes, all the other remaining diseases show symptoms, which disturb vision.

In general, the tablet BM 54641+ fits well into the tradition of medical texts about eye diseases as known from cuneiform texts from Assyria and Babylonia from the Middle Assyrian until the Late Babylonian period. The structure of the tablet – the entries are organized according to the symptoms – and identical prescriptions prove the background was at least a similar. This is by no means surprising, if one considers the large

[25] See Fincke, *Augenleiden*, 86–91.

[26] Compare however the different interpretation of the relevant cuneiform signs by JoAnn Scurlock, for this see above footnote 23.

number of tablets that, according to their colophons, Assyrian scholars copied from tablets from Borsippa[27] and other Babylonian cities.

BM 40737

This fragment[28] is 6.4 cm wide, 3.7 cm high, and 0.23 cm thick. It comes from Babylonia, but is of otherwise unknown provenance, and might well be a school-tablet. Not one prescription has a parallel in any other known medical text, so it is difficult to establish how much of the tablet is missing, and the shape of the edges does not help in this respect.

obv.

1′ [__ __ _]_ [
2′ [K]I.⸢MIN⸣ NA$_4$.*mu-ṣa* KI.MIN N[A$_4$.
3′ 1 NA$_4$.MUŠ.⸢GÍR KI⸣.MIN ⸢__ KI$^{?}$⸣.M[IN$^{?}$
4′ *ina* Ì KUR.GI.MUŠEN KI.MIN ⸢__ KI$^{?}$.MIN$^{?}$ __⸣ _[_

5′ DIŠ NA IGI^{II}-*šú* ÚŠ ⸢SA$_5$⸣ U$_5$.GAR.IB.⸢MUŠEN *ina*⸣ _[_

6′ Ì.UDU ⸢*kur*⸣-*sin-na-a-tú* UDU NÍTA ⸢*šá* ŠE.MAŠ$^{?}$⸣ *lu* Ì.UDU *šá* GIŠ.⸢__⸣.[
7′ *ina* GU.ZI (read: GÚ.ZI) *ina* UGU RU-UN-ṬU GAR-*an* ⸢DUḪ.LÀL⸣ IB-⸢__⸣-[
8′ *bit-qa gu-uḫ-lu šá e-du-*⸢*um ina* ŠÀ⸣ SÚD IGI^{II}-*š*[*ú tuṣammid*
9′ NA$_4$.*as-ḫar ba-šal ina* ŠÀ-*bi* SÚD IGI^{II}-*šú* MAR.MEŠ-*m*[*a*

rev.

1 *me-su-ú ina* ŠÀ-*bi* ⸢SÚD⸣ IGI^{II}-*šú* MAR.MEŠ-*ma* ZI *ki-i* _[_
2 SÚD IGI^{II}-*šú* MAR.MEŠ-*ma* ZI *ana* IGI *šá* IGI *i-kaš-š*[*ad*

---

3 DIŠ NA IGI^{II} *šá* ⸢LÚ⸣.TUR KI.MIN *ma-la te-qít* K[A
4 *lu šá bir-rat* IGI^{II} *lu šá a-mur-din-nu šá* IG[I^{II}
5 *šá* LA$^{?}$ Ú.ḪI.A *ar*$^{!?}$(RI)-*qud-su* MAR.MEŠ _[_

---

6 [DIŠ KI.MI]N *gu-ḫúl šá i-du-um* [
7 [__ __ _]_ 2 GÍN *ṣa-di-di*_[_
8 (traces)
(rest of reverse is missing)

[27] See H. Hunger, *Babylonische und assyrische Kolophone*, Alter Orient und Altes Testament 2 (Neukirchen-Vluyn: Verlag Butzon & Bercker Kevelaer, 1968), 157 (index for Borsippa).

[28] In 2005, Christopher B.F. Walker kindly allowed me to use the database he had created for the future volumes of the *Catalogue of the Babylonian Tablets in the British Museum*, from which I located this tablet.

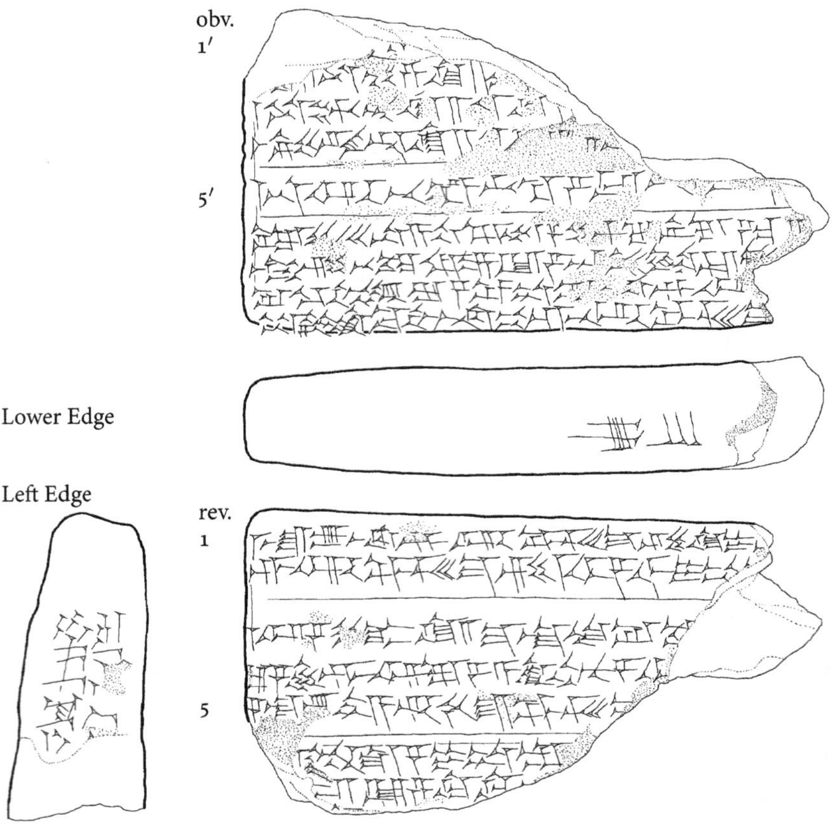

Figure 3: BM 40737
(See corresponding figure 6; page 104)

lower edge

1 [...] 3-*ú*[29]

left edge

1 GIM ⌜SUMUN⌝-*šú* [
2 IM ^{m}*bul-luṭ*-[

---

[29] Written in the opposite direction to the lines of obverse and reverse.

Translation:

obv.

1′ (traces)
2′ [di]tto; *mūṣu*-mineral ditto; [...-mine]ral [ditto; ...]
3′ 1 *muššaru*-mineral ditto; ... [...]
4′ in fat of a goose ditto; ... [...]

5′ If someone's eyes are full of blood: "spur of a bat"-drug in ..[... ...]

6′ Fat from the ankle of a (male) sheep that was (fed with) barley or fat from ..[... ...]
7′ you place in a cup! on top of a *runṭu*, wax .. [...]
8′ You grind 1/8 shekel of antimony from Edom (and) hi[s] eyes [*you bandage.* ...]
9′ cooked! *asḫar*-mineral you grind inside (or: into it), daub his eyes, an[d ...]

rev.

1 *mēsu*-tree you grind inside (or: into it), daub his eyes, and ZI like ..[... ...]
2 you grind, daub his eyes, and ZI will arrive at the front of the eye (?) [...]

---

3 If the eyes of a child are ditto: equivalent to the ointment ..[...]
4 either for *birratu* of the eyes or for *amurdinnu* of the eye[s...]
5 of leaves of plants – in their greenness – you daub, ..[...]

---

6 [If ditt]o: antimony from Edom [...]
7 [..]. 2 shekel of *ṣadīdu*-antimony ..[...]
8 (traces)
(rest of reverse is missing)

lower edge

1 [...] third.

left edge

1 According to its original [...]
2 Tablet of Bulluṭ-[...]

Commentary:

obv. 1′–4′

The first prescription uses various stones all processed in the same way. According to line 4′, one ingredient that is not known to us will be used together with "fat of a goose" in the same way. This suggests that all ingredients will be ground.

obv. 5′

The second prescription deals with blood in the eye. In this case, the drug called "spur of a bat" is the main component to be ground or mixed with another ingredient; according to other texts this could be either some kind of fat or honey. "Spur of a bat"-drug is regularly used in the treatment of eyes.

obv. 6′–rev. 2

The third prescription runs over from the obverse to the reverse of the tablet. Although there is no reference to any previous symptom (DIŠ KI.MIN "If ditto"), it may still be dealing with blood in the eye. This prescription includes some uncommon instructions, as well as being very difficult to read, so a comment on each single line is called for:

Line 6′ is easy to understand, although its content has no parallel among the other medical texts on eye diseases.

In line 7′, the scribe made at least two mistakes. At the beginning of the line, he wrote GU.ZI instead of GÚ.ZI for *kāsu* "cup". What the scribe meant by writing RU-UN-ṬU is not clear. At the end of this line, DUḪ.LÀL IB-x seems to be an appropriate reading, because other medical texts have DUḪ.LÀL (*iškūra*) *lā balla* "unmixed wax". It would be nice to restore a form from *balālu* "to mix", but the traces of the following cuneiform signs make no sense. The translation given above seems the best proposal.

In line 8′ there is a reference to *guḫlû ša edum* "antimony from Edom", as also in reverse, line 6, where it is written: *gu-ḫúl šá i-du-um*.

Antimony from Edom had a certain quality. At the beginning of the 7th century B.C. antimony[30] from that region formed part of the tribute Sennacherib received from Hezekiah, king of Judah. For many years, Edom was more or less controlled by Judah. Antimony from Edom is also mentioned in Finkel, FS Lambert, no. 22A (BM 42638+) obv. 6: [... *gu*]-*uḫ-lu*₄ *šá* KUR.*i-du-um-mu in* LÀL IGI-*a-šú tu*-LAL "[... with ... (and) ant]imony from Edom (mixed) with honey you bandage his eyes".[31] This is one of the Late Babylonian school-tablets from Sippar that

[30] For antimony see P.R.S. Moorey, *Materials and Manufacture in Ancient Mesopotamia: The Evidence of Archaeology and Art. Metals and Metalwork, Glazed Materials and Glass*, BAR International Series 237 (Oxford: John and Erika Hedge Ltd, 1985), 1–4.

[31] I would like to thank Irving L. Finkel for this reference.

deals with eye diseases. It opens up the possibility of restoring *tuṣammid* 'you bandage' at the end of line 8′.

In line 9′, the scribe made another mistake by writing *asḫar ba-šal* instead of *asḫar bašla*, "cooked *asḫar*-mineral". He must have interpreted NA4.*as-ḫar* as *status constructus* and formed the adjective accordingly.

In rev. lines 1 and 2, the sign ZI seems to represent a kind of disease or symptom. Because the scribe wrote a logogram already incorrectly in line 7′, it could be that here the sign ZI is a mistake for SI, *qarnu* "horn". If so, it could mean a kind of "splinter" had entered the eye. For the moment the sign is just transliterated, not translated.

rev. 3–5

This prescription for a child's symptom is otherwise unknown. Medication appropriate for *birratu* or *amurdinnu* of the eyes is to be used (see line 4). According to the series "If someone's eyes are diseased", both *birratu* and *amurdinnu* are symptoms associated with strong irritation in the eyes, but the exact meaning of these words in this context is not known.[32]

rev. 6–7

The last prescription of this fragment uses antimony from Edom, mentioned earlier in obv. 8′, and *ṣadīdu*-antimony, mentioned only in one other medical text on eye diseases (BM 132097), the Neo-Babylonian tablet of unknown provenance, a prescription on which begins (8′): [...N]A4.*aš-gì-gì* NA4.UGU-*aš-gì-gì* NA4.*ṣa-di-di* (9′) [... ŠU]M-*aḫ* ... '[...] *ašgikû*-mineral, *eli-ašgikû*-mineral, *ṣadīdu*-antimony [... you sc]atter;[33] ...'

lower edge 1, left edge 1–2

The beginning of the colophon on the lower edge 3, 3-*ú*, presumably indicates that the tablet is the third one of a series on eye diseases. But the phonetic complement -*ú* would be correct only for *šanû* (the second tablet) or *rebû* (the fourth one). It can be considered a mistake for 3.KAM. The rest of the colophon is written on the left edge, and confirms that the tablet was a copy *kīma labirī-šu* [....] 'according to its original [...]'. The name of the scribe begins with the element Bulluṭ-[...].

---

32 See Fincke, *Augenleiden*, 86–91, 192–193.

33 ŠUM, *ṭabāḫu* 'to slaughter' is to be interpreted as *sapāḫu* 'to scatter, to disperse' in this context, see E. von Weiher, *Spätbabylonische Texte aus Uruk*, II, Ausgrabungen der Deutschen Forschungsgemeinschaft in Uruk-Warka 9 (Berlin: Gebr. Mann, 1976), 195–196 commentary to line 3.

Orientation of Late Babylonian School-Tablets

Because BM 40737 does seem to be a school-tablet, it should be compared with the Late Babylonian school-tablets of the Sippar archive, which were examined by Finkel. He found that tablets with therapeutic treatments that are commonly thought to belong to the "profession of a physician" (*asûtu*) were written with landscape orientation, whereas the tablets with instructions for rituals and incantations, the magico-medical tablets, which belonged to those concerned with "exorcism" (*āšipūtu*), were written with horizontal orientation.[34] An examination of the Neo- and Late Babylonian medical texts on eye diseases shows that they were oriented in both ways.

Medical texts on eye diseases	**Landscape orientation**	**Portrait orientation**	**Unknown orientation**
Neo-Babylonian:	BAM IV 382	BM 54641 + 54826 Geller, AfO 35, 22–23	BM 40737
Late Babylonian:	Finkel FS Lambert no. 12 Finkel FS Lambert no. 22	SpTU II 50	BAM IV 410

Apart from the Late Babylonian texts published by Finkel, only the Neo-Babylonian tablet BAM IV 382 fits into Finkel's scheme. The other Neo- and Late Babylonian tablets show either portrait (three tablets) or unknown orientation (two tablets). These texts from the first millennium B.C. neither support nor disprove the assumption that the orientation of the tablets is connected with the profession of *asûtu* or *āšipūtu*. It could be that such a division is only true for school-tablets, for school-tablets from Babylonia, or even for school-tablets only from Sippar.

34 Finkel, FS Lambert, 146.

Table 1. ***Sequence of Symptoms Within the Series DIŠ NA IGI^{II}-šú GIG 'if someone's eyes are diseased'***

1. **tablet** col. i-iii 1. tablet col. iv	'red eye'	– 'blood' in the eye (ÚŠ, *dāmu*)
2. **tablet** col. i	foreign bodies	– real foreign bodies
		– sty, hordeolum (*merḫu ša īni*)
		– secretions of various origin (*lipištu*, ...)
		– hair (SÍK *aṣât* "a hair grows (out of the eye)")
		– "swelling of conjunctiva" (UZU *āliku*, *šīru āliku*)
		– membranes (*šišītu*)
		– etc.
2. tablet col. i-ii	dysfunction of lachrymal gland	– too many tears, *epiphoria* (ÉR, *dimtu*)
		– not enough tears, (DIŠ NA IGI^{II}-*šú* ḪÁD.DA GIG, *īnā-šu tābīla marṣā*)
2. tablet col. ii	eye lids	– disease of eye lids (GIG.GIR, *k/gurāru*)
2. tablet col. ii	inside of the eye	– icterus (IGI.SIG$_7$.SIG$_7$, *amurriqānu ša īnī*)
		– 'membranes and shadow' (*šišītu* and GISSU)
2. tablet col. ii–iii	eyesight	– bad eyesight (*digil-šu kabit* 'his eyesight is bad')
2. tablet col. iii–iv	'shadow'	– 'shadow' (GISSU, *ṣillu*)
3. **tablet** col. i	vision	– photopsia, a main symptom of 'hand of a ghost' (ŠU-GIDIM.MA)
3. tablet col. ii	eyesight	– sudden blindness
	vision	– seeing double, diplopia (*digil īnī-šu mādi*, 'the vision of his eyes is numerous')[35]
	eyesight	– blindness
		– night/day blindness (*sîn-lurmâ*)
3. tablet col. iii–iv	not preserved	

[35] Scurlock, *Diagnosis*, 187 § 9.7 reads the relevant passsage differently: DIŠ NA IGI^{II}-*šú ma-a-ṭi* "If a person's eyesight is diminished ..."

Table 2. BM 54641 + 54826: Symptoms

obv. 1′–2′	[DIŠ NA IGI^{II}-*šú* UZU DU-*ka* SI.A.MEŠ] ?	[If someone's eyes are full of growing / moving flesh] ?	= BAM I 22 obv. 4′–8′?, and BAM VI 515 ii 22′–24′ ?
obv. 3′–4′	[DIŠ NA IGI^{II}-*šú*] ⸢UZU *u* ÚŠ⸣ S[I].⸢A⸣.MEŠ	[If someone's eyes] are full of flesh and blood	= BAM I 22 obv. 9′–11′
obv. 5′	[DIŠ NA IG]I^{II}-*šú* ÚŠ ⸢SI.A⸣.[MEŠ]	[If someone's ey]es are full of blood	
obv. 6′–7′	[DIŠ NA IGI^{II}-*šú* Ú]Š SI.A.MEŠ-*ma* x[x ...]	[If someone's eyes] are full of blood and .[...]	
obv. 8′–12′	⸢DIŠ NA IGI⸣[^{II}-*šú* ÚŠ] SI.A.MEŠ *ur-ri u* GE$_6$ *la* ⸢*i*⸣-[*ṣ*]*a-lal-*⸢*ma la ina-ṭal é*$^?$⸣-*kil* IGI^{II}-⸢*šú*⸣ [__ __] / ŠÀ I[GI^{II}-*šú*] SA$_5$.MEŠ IGI^{II}-*šú* DUL-*ma*	If someone's ey[s] are full of [blood], day and night he cannot sleep, and he cannot see; the dark (part)$^?$ of his eyes [...], / the inside of [his] e[yes] is (completely) red (and) his eyes are covered	= BAM VI 510 i 31′–34′ // 513 i 21′–25′ // 514 i 38′–42′
obv. 13′	DIŠ NA [IGI^{II} KI.MIN]	If someone's [eyes are ditto]	
obv. 14′	DIŠ N[A IGI^{II}-*šú* ÚŠ *šu-u*]*n-n*[*u-ʾa*]	If someo[ne's eyes are bl]ock[ed with blood]	= BAM I 18 obv. 1–2, and BAM VI 513 i 26′ // 514 i 43′
obv. 15′	[DIŠ NA] I[GI^{II}]-⸢*šú*⸣ [Ú]Š *iṭ-ri-ma* GUB-*iz*	[If bl]ood penetrates [someone]'s e[yes] and it stays	similar to BAM I 22 rev. 25′–26′
obv. 16′–18′	[DIŠ NA] IGI^{II}-*šú* *šik-*⸢*na šá* ÚŠ⸣ *š*[*ak-n*]*a*	[If someone's] eyes have a layer of blood	similar to BAM I 22 rev. 27′–31′, and to BAM VI 513 ii 13′–15′ // 514 ii 9′–11′
obv. 19′–20′	DIŠ NA IGI^{II}-*šú* ⸢*i*⸣-[*bar-ru*]-⸢*ra*⸣	If someone's eyes *ibarrurā*	= SpTU II 50 obv. 15– rev. 1
rev. 1	DIŠ KI.MIN	If ditto	= BAM II 159 iv 26′–27′
rev. 2–3	DIŠ KI.MIN	If ditto	similar to BAM II 159 iv 23′–24′, and to SpTU II 50 obv. 10–13

rev. 4	[DIŠ NA] ⌜IGI⌝^{II}-*šú* *i-bar-ru-r*[*a ù* É]R ⌜*ú-kal*⌝-*la*	[If someone's] eyes *ibarrurā* [and] hold [te]ars	= SpTU II 50 rev. 18 ; similar to BAM II 159 iv 28′–29′
rev. 5	⌜DIŠ NA IGI^{II}-*šú* ÉR SI.A⌝.[MEŠ]	If someone's eyes are full of tears	= BAM II 159 v 1–2 ?
rev. 6–7	DIŠ NA IGI^{II}-*šú* ÉR *im-l*[*a*?-*a*]	If someone's eyes fill up with tears	
rev. 8	DIŠ NA IGI^{II}-*šú* *lu* ÉR (over erasure) ⌜*lu* ZÁḪ⌝ ŠUB.ŠUB.A	If someone's eyes are thrown either into tears or into 'lost'	= BAM II 159 v 3–4
rev. 9	[DIŠ N]A IGI^{II}-*šú* LÙ.LÙ-⌜*ḫa*⌝	[If some]one's eyes are constantly blurred	= SpTU II 50 rev. 24
rev. 10	[DIŠ NA IG]I^{II}-*šú* *ri-šu*-⌜*ta*$_5$⌝ SI.A.MEŠ	[If someone's ey]es are full of redness	
rev. 11–12	[DIŠ NA IGI^{I}]^{I}-⌜*šú* *i*⌝-*pi*-⌜*ta*$_5$⌝ *bir-ra-ta*$_5$ *u* *gu-qa-na ú-kal-la*	[If someone's eyes] hold "clouding over", *birratu* or *qūqānu*	
rev. 13–18	[DIŠ NA IGI^{II}-*šú* *bir-r*]*a-ta*$_5$ *a-šá-a* SA$_5$.⌜MEŠ⌝	[If someone's eyes] are troubled because of [*birr*]*atu* (and) are red	

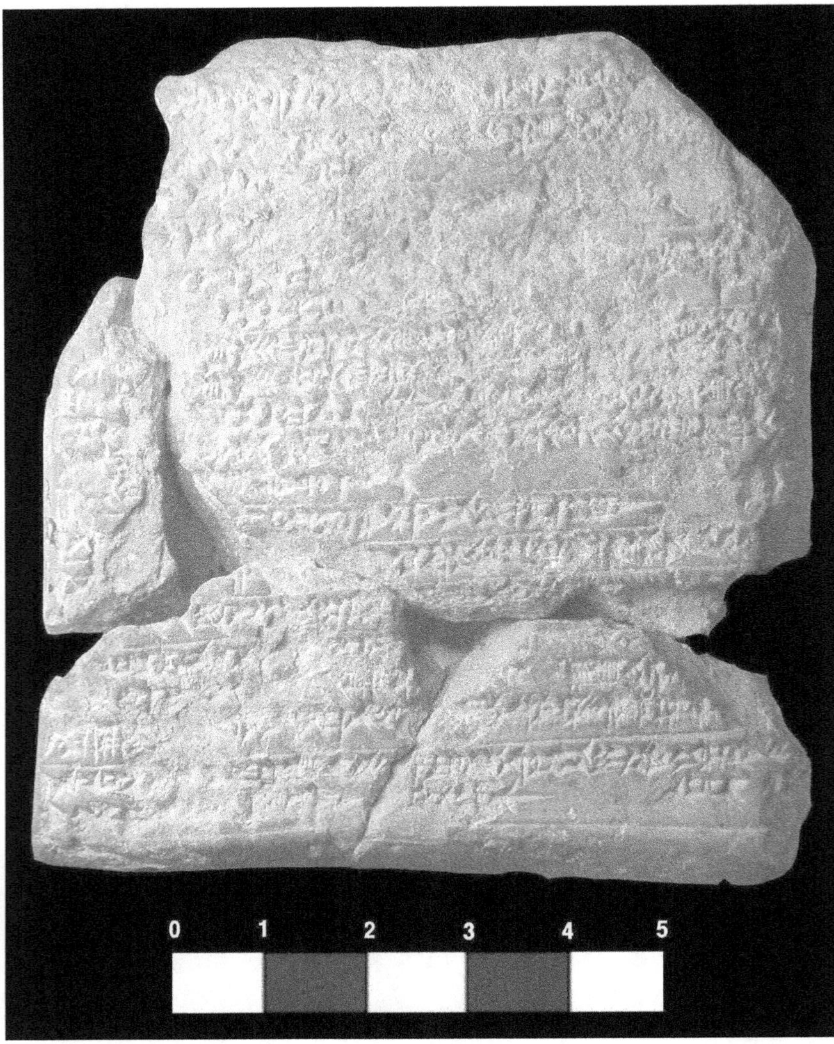

Figure 4: BM 54641+ obverse

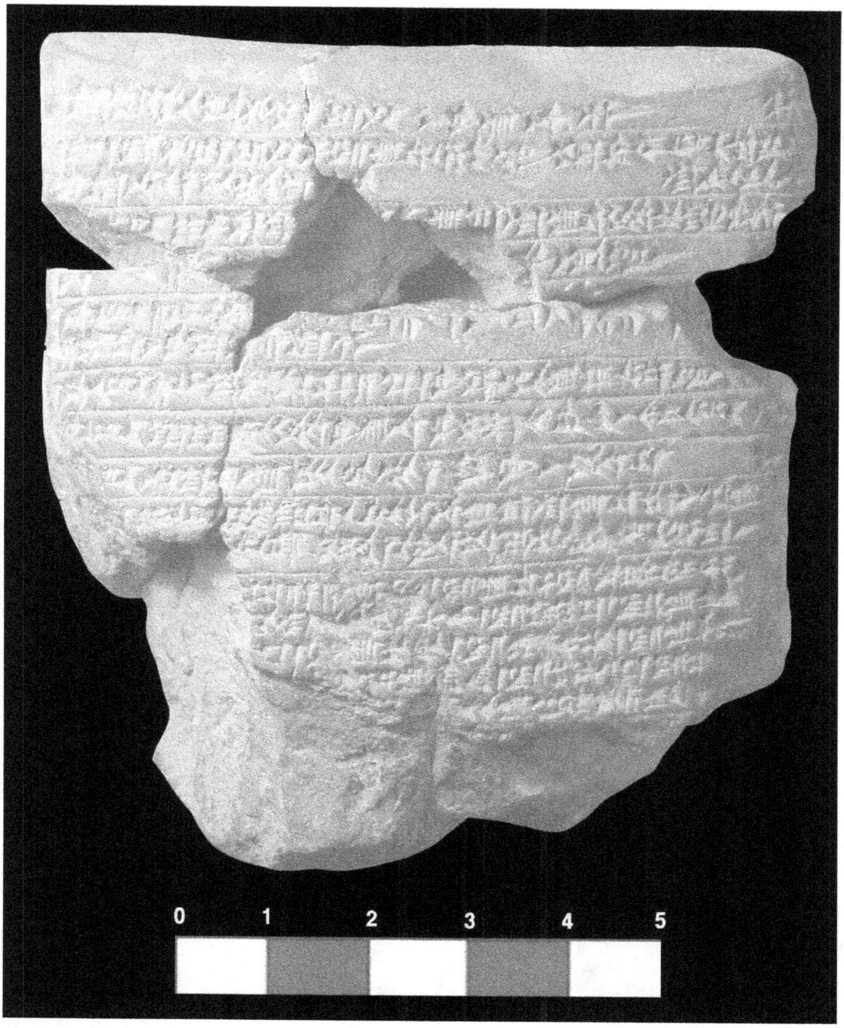

Figure 5: BM 54641+ reverse

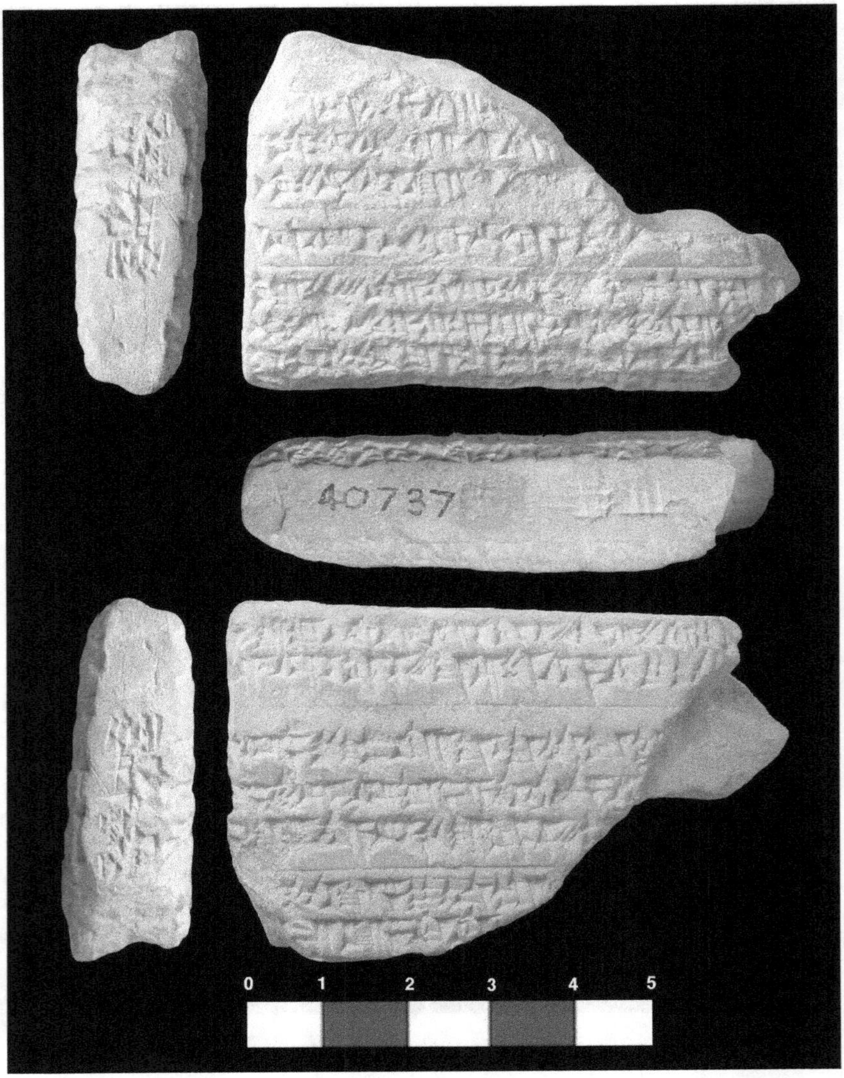

Figure 6: BM 40737

ON MEDICAL TECHNOLOGY IN ANCIENT MESOPOTAMIA

BARBARA BÖCK*

1. *Introduction*

As is well known, the corpus of medical texts falls into three major groups: (a) Characteristic of the first group is the connection between symptoms of diseases and their respective prognosis. These texts, which are generally labelled prognostic-diagnostic, do not only predict the outcome of a set of symptoms – recovery or death of the patient – but also attribute the disorder to the realm of the supernatural.[1] (b) Similar in

* Instituto de Lenguas y Culturas del Mediterráneo y Oriente Próximo, CSIC, Madrid, barbara.boeck@cchs.csic.es. This work has been supported by the Spanish Government, MEC, HUM2005-007 35/FILO. I wish to thank the editors for reading and making suggestions on an earlier draft of the paper.

[1] The *editio princeps* is that of the René Labat, *Traité akkadien de diagnostics et pronostics médicaux*, 2 volumes (Paris: E.J. Brill, 1951); additional texts have been published by Marten Stol, *Epilepsy in Babylonia* (Groningen: Styx Publication, 1993), 56–98; the Akkadian tradition at the Hittite capital has been studied by Gernot Wilhelm, *Medizinische Omina aus Ḫattuša ina akkadischer Sprache* (Wiesbaden: Harrassowitz Verlag, 1994); a work to complement Labat's edition has been offered by Nils Heeßel, *Babylonisch-assyrische Diagnostik*, Alter Orient und Altes Testament 43 (Münster: Ugarit Verlag, 2000). For an attempt to identify ancient Mesopotamian diseases see the work of JoAnn Scurlock and Burton R. Andersen, *Diagnoses in Assyrian and Babylonian Medicine* (Urbana/Chicago: University of Illinois Press, 2005).

The following abbreviations of text editions have been used: *AMT* = Reginald Campbell Thompson, *Assyrian Medical Texts*, (London/Oxford: Clarendon Press, 1923); *BAM* = Franz Köcher, *Die Babylonisch-assyrische Medizin in Texten und Untersuchungen*, vols. I–VI, (Berlin: Walter de Gruyter & Co, 1963–1980); *CT* = *Cuneiform Texts from Babylonian Tablets in the British Museum*, vol. 4: Thompson, (London: Harrison & Son, 1902); *CT* 23: Thompson (London: Harrison and Sons, 1906); *KADP* = Franz Köcher, *Keilschrifttexte zur assyrisch-babylonischen Drogen- und Pflanzenkunde* (Berlin: Akademie-Verlag, 1955); *KAR* = Erich Ebeling, *Keilschrifttexte aus Assur religiösen Inhalts*, (Leipzig: J.C. Hinrichs'sche Buchhandlung, 1915–1923 [= *Wissenschaftliche Veröffentlichungen der Deutschen Orient-Gesellschaft* vol. 28, 34]); *KUB* = *Keilschrifturkunden aus Boghazköy*, vol. 4: Ernst Weidner, (Berlin: Akademie-Verlag, 1922); *KUB* vol. 37: Franz Köcher

content as far as the description of symptoms is concerned are therapeutic or recipe texts which give detailed information about preparing and administering a variety of remedies, usually based on medicinal plants.[2] (c) The third group of texts, namely those of pharmaceutical content, is quite heterogeneous. Here, one may distinguish between three subgroups: plant-description texts similar in structure to the famous compendium of Dioscorides (but lacking images), lists of simple drugs and the encyclopaedic handbook of drugs Uruanna.[3]

The vast numbers of cuneiform texts were grouped together and arranged in antiquity according to content. Like the majority of ancient Mesopotamian literature, medical texts were standardized and compiled into handbooks with a title and an established sequence of chapters. It is generally agreed that this process took place as early as the third quarter of the second millennium B.C.[4]

The result of the standardization is evident in texts and fragments dating to the first millennium B.C. As far as the handbook of prescriptions is concerned, we see it best in the copy from Ashurbanipal's palace library at Nineveh. As is well known, this Assyrian king who reigned from 668 to 627 B.C. ordered the collection, confiscation and compilation of nearly all the literary cuneiform output and completed the library project

(Berlin: Akademie-Verlag, 1953); *STT* I = Oliver R. Gurney / Jacob J. Finkelstein, *The Sultantepe Tablets* I, (London/Bradford: Percy Lund, Humphries and Company Ltd., 1957), *STT* II = Gurney / Peter Hulin (London/Bradford: Percy Lund, Humphries and Company Ltd., 1964). The two main dictionaries of the Akkadian language are *AHw* = Wolfram von Soden, *Akkadisches Handwörterbuch*, vol. I–III (Wiesbaden: Otto Harrassowitz, 1965–1981), and *CAD* = *The Chicago Assyrian Dictionary*, vol. 1–21 (Chicago: J.J. Augustin Verlagsbuchhandlung, Glückstadt, and Winona Lake, IN: Eisenbrauns, 1956–).

[2] The edition of remedies is closely linked to the names of Reginald Campbell Thompson (e.g. *CT* 23, *AMT*) and Franz Köcher (*BAM* I–VI).

[3] The critical edition and study of pharmaceutical texts was the lifetime project of the assyriologist and historian of ancient medicine Franz Köcher. The relevant text material, which was found in the city of Ashur, is published in autography in his volume *KADP*; for texts from Nineveh see the edition of cuneiform copies by Thompson, *CT* 14. After the death of Franz Köcher in 2002, the completion, edition and study of all pertinent texts is now the task of the present author. Some features of the handbook Uruanna: *maštakal*, which enumerates in two columns medicinal plants and other *materia medica*, have been recently discussed by James V. Kinnier Wilson in his contribution "The Assyrian Pharmaceutical Series URU.AN.NA: *maštakal*," *Journal of Near Eastern Studies* 64 (2005): 45–51.

[4] For the process of standardization see A. Leo Oppenheim, *Ancient Mesopotamia. Portrait of a Dead Civilization* (Chicago/London: The University of Chicago Press, 1977), 18.

that had already been initiated by his father, Esarhaddon.[5] Similar to other text genres of scholarly tradition complementary medical literature developed ranging from various kinds of commentaries up to entire sets of excerpt (Akk. *nisḫu*) and section (Akk. *pirsu*) series with their own chapter numeration. However, not all recipes formed part of handbooks. As is stated in colophons from texts found at Assur, very often the practitioner would make an excerpt just for *ad hoc* use. Other texts represent in all likelihood exercise tablets of apprentices, as suggested by an archive coming from Sippar.[6]

The handbook of remedies which forms the basis for the present study is structured according to the common scheme listing the prescriptions thematically *a capite ad calcem*. It was known in antiquity under the title "If the upper part of a man's head is hot" and contained at least 45 chapters, which were thematically grouped together into bigger units each provided with a "subtitle" and an independent chapter numeration. So we find, for example, a unit of remedies against eye diseases entitled "If a man suffers from pain in the eyes" that contains three chapters each of approximately 50 to 60 recipes, another unit with prescriptions against diseases connected with the nose and breathing called "If a man's nose (breath) is heavy" and containing six chapters, a third unit of recipes for renal diseases known as "If a man's kidneys cause him constantly pain" with three chapters, etc.[7]

---

[5] Administrative records, which state the genesis of Assurbanipal's library have been studied by Simo Parpola, "Assyrian Library Records," *Journal of Near Eastern Studies* 42 (1983): 1–29. Colophons that refer to the Assyrian king as a scribe have been published by Hermann Hunger, *Babylonische und assyrische Kolophone*, Alter Orient und Altes Testament 2 (Neukirchen-Vluyn: Verlag Butzon & Bercker Kevelaer, 1968), 97–106 (nos. 318, 319, 321, 323–325, 327–330, 337–338). For a study of Ashurbanipal's library see Stephen J. Lieberman, "Canonical and official cuneiform texts: Towards an understanding of Assurbanipal's personal tablet collection," in *Lingering over Words. Studies in Ancient Near Eastern Literature in Honor of William L. Moran*, eds. Tzvi Abusch et al. (Atlanta: Scholar's Press, 1990), 305–336. On the formation of the royal libraries at Nineveh see also the contribution of Grant Frame and Andrew R. George, "The Royal Libraries of Nineveh: New Evidence for King Ashurbanipal's Tablet Collecting," *Iraq* 67 (2005): 265–284.

[6] The colophons from some of the tablets unearthed at Ashur have been treated by Hunger, *Babylonische und assyrische Kolophone*; for colophons stating the quick excerpting of prescriptions see e.g. nos. 197, 201, 202, and 208. The medical texts coming from an archive in Sippar have been studied by Irving L. Finkel, "On Late Babylonian Medical Training," in *Wisdom, Gods and Literature. Studies in Assyriology in Honour of W.G. Lambert*, eds. A.R. George and I.L. Finkel, (Winona Lake, IN: Eisenbrauns, 2000), 137–223.

[7] See the discussion of Köcher "Spätbabylonische Texte aus Uruk," in *Medizinische Diagnostik in Geschichte und Gegenwart*, C. Habrich et al. eds. (Munich: Werner Fritsch,

The remedies offer a remarkable insight into many facets of Babylonian and Assyrian healing therapies. Since the study and discussion of healing methods has tended to focus on magical practices[8] the general impression of ancient Mesopotamian medicine is that the efficacy of therapies depends to a great extent on symbolic manipulation and ritual performance. This assessment is, of course, not to be dismissed, but should be modified. Analysing the text material, it becomes clear that both concepts – ritual act and material effect – are more often than not intertwined.

Nevertheless, if we try to separate magic from science, we can distinguish between different techniques of drug extraction while preparing medicaments. Now, we can never be positive about whether the ancient practitioner used and deliberately preferred one extraction method to another, depending, for instance, on the family of the medicinal plant in question or its respective part such as seeds, fruits, roots, stems, or leaves. Another issue that seriously hampers our understanding of the therapeutic effect of healing therapies is the identification of ancient Mesopotamian medicinal plants. This obstacle does not only apply to medicinal plants but also to ancient Mesopotamian vegetation in general, including food plants.

In spite of fundamental studies such as Immanuel Löw's *Die Flora der Juden*,[9] Reginald Campbell Thompson's *A Dictionary of Assyrian Botany*,[10] and a number of individual studies such as the contributions published in volumes 2 and 3 of the *Bulletin on Sumerian Agriculture*,[11] the relevant literature, especially the modern dictionaries of Akkadian language, are filled with contradictions and speculations. As one example one may refer to the plant called in Akkadian *saḫlû*, identifications of

1978), 17–39, 18–20. For eye diseases see also the references given by Köcher in *BAM* VI, ix–xiv; for diseases affecting the respiration see Köcher *BAM* VI, xxi–xxv; and for the unit on kidney diseases see Markham J. Geller, *Renal and Rectal Disease Texts, Die babylonisch-assyrische Medizin* 7 (Berlin/New York: Walter de Gruyter, 2005).

[8] See for example the studies of Walter Farber, *Beschwörungsrituale an Ištar und Dumuzi* (Wiesbaden: Franz Steiner Verlag, 1977); Daniel Schwemer, *Akkadische Rituale aus Ḫattuša* (Heidelberg: Universitätsverlag C. Winter, 1998); Erica Reiner, *Astral Magic in Babylonia* (Philadelphia: The American Philosophical Society, 1995), 43–60.

[9] 4 volumes (Vienna/Leipzig: R. Löwit, 1924–1934), re-printed (Hildesheim: Georg Olms Verlagsbuchhandlung, 1967).

[10] (London: Stephen Austin and Sons, Ltd., 1949). Thompson's work was made available posthumously by his wife, Barbara Campbell Thompson.

[11] Vol. II of the *Bulletin on Sumerian Agriculture* (1985) is dedicated to legumes and oil seed-crops, and vol. III (1987), to onions, cucumbers, and fruit trees.

which include watercress, cardamom, and wolfberry.[12] However, none of these suggestions takes into account its appearance as portrayed in the plant description text "On the nature of the medicinal plant" (Akk. *šammu šikinšu*). One of the main characteristics of the plant, namely that it has thorns or a hooked and barbed surface (the Akkadian term used here – *kakku*, literally "weapon" – is ambiguous) is a feature that is clearly not typical of either of the given identifications.[13] As has been recently stressed:

> Species identification must always proceed from etymology to a consideration of context, with an awareness of the history of the flora in the region (including the Mediterranean) and of the evidence of archeobotany. If the etymological and other evidence agrees, then probable solutions become possible. However, where the linguistic evidence is confused or ambivalent (...) it may never, given the nature of what is normally recorded in cuneiform sources, be possible to arrive at satisfactory identifications.[14]

Accordingly, in what follows we shall use the Akkadian plant name and give identifications only if reasonable.

This introduction would not be complete without a short note on the long debate about the responsibilities of the two medical professions. It has often been argued that diseases falling into the supernatural realm are to be treated by the "incantation priest" (Akk. *āšipu*), whereas the cure of less serious disorders, minor surgical interventions, or collecting herbs were entrusted to the medical practitioner called in Akk. *asû* ("practical doctor"). Nevertheless, neither the information given in the recipes nor what appears in the colophons of medical texts allow for such a distinction. Likewise, the characterisation of the *asû* as pharmacist or herb

---

[12] See the discussion of Franz Köcher "Ein Text medizinischen Inhalts aus dem neubabylonischen Grab 405," in *Uruk; Die Gräber*, eds. R.M. Boehmer et al., Ausgrabungen in Uruk-Warka, 10 (Mainz: Philipp von Zabern, 1995), 203–217, 212. See the discussion by Marvin A. Powell, "Obst und Gemüse. A.I," *Reallexikon für Assyriologie und Vorderasiatische Altertumskunde* 10 (2003): 13–22, on pp. 14–15. For the identification of *saḫlû* with garden cress see Benno Landsberger, "Zur Mehlbereitung im Altertum," *Orientalistische Literaturzeitung* 25, (1922): 387–344, 343 fn. 3). Since the Greek term for garden cress is κάρδαμον, which also stands for cardamom, the two plants seem to have been confused. Thompson, for example, in his *A Dictionary of Assyrian Botany*, (London: the British Academy, 1949), 58 speaks of "*saḫlû* (...) the seed of the ordinary cardamon, cress." For the identification with wolfberry see Volkert Haas, *Materia magica et medica hethitica* (Berlin/New York: Walter de Gruyter, 2003), 2 vols., 349–350.

[13] The text in question is published as *KADP* 33. The *saḫlû* plant appears as *tertium comparationis* in obv. 12: *šammu šikin-šú kakkī-šú kīma kakki saḫlê*, "The appearance of the officinal plant (is as follows): its 'thorns' are like the 'thorns' of the *saḫlû* plant."

[14] Powell, "Obst und Gemüse," *Reallexikon für Assyriologie* 10, (2003–5): 15.

collector[15] should rather be modified, since many of the pharmacological texts such as the handbook URU.AN.NA: *maštakal* are connected with the incantation priest.[16] As a working hypothesis, we propose that the prescriptions represent the know-how as well as the experience of both practitioners. The compilation and redaction of the texts into handbooks and compendia, however, should be assigned to the incantation priest.[17]

2. *Methods of Drug Extraction*

Contrary to Greek or Latin medical tradition in classical antiquity ancient Mesopotamian scholarship did not produce any theoretical work or treatise. Babylonian and Assyrian practitioners did not summarize recipes according to preparation and application but rather stated how drugs were prepared and administered in each remedy in a somewhat casuistic manner. The descriptions range from brief sketches to more elaborate explanations. It is not clear what the motives are for shorter or longer versions: supposed degree of knowledge, individual style, or limit of time when copying and formulating a recipe.

Many plants used for the preparation of remedies were dried. Though seldom explicitly stated, this is evident from additional expressions when fresh ingredients were occasionally required (in Akk. we find the designation *(w)arqūssu* "(in) its green state" following the plant), or when the substances in question would still need to be dried for further preparation (in Akk. formulated *tubbal* "you shall dry"). Sometimes a reference is given to the place where the drug was dried, namely in the shadow, or the

15 As stated by JoAnn Scurlock in her contribution "Physician, Exorcist, Conjurer, Magician: A Tale of Two Healing Professionals", in *Mesopotamian Magic: Textual, Historical, and Interpretative Perspectives*, eds. T. Abusch and K. van der Toorn, Ancient Magic and Divination 1 (Groningen: Styx Publications 1999), 69–79, p. 79.

16 *Pace* JoAnn Scurlock "Physician, Exorcist, Conjurer, Magician", 75. A copy of URU.AN.NA: *maštakal* from Nimrud (published as *CTN* IV 192) is identified as a "tablet of Banuni, the incantation priest"; further examples are *KADP* 2 or *KADP* 4 which were both found in the library N4 belonging to the family of the incantation priests Baba-šuma-ibni, Nabû-bēssunu, Kiṣir-Aššur and Kiṣir-Nabû (cf. Olof Pedersén, *Archives and Libraries in the City of Assur. A Survey of the Material from the German Excavations* II (Uppsala: Acta Universitatis Upsaliensis, 1986), p. 71, 68).

17 For a discussion of the relevant literature see my contribution "Heilkundige und Heilkunst im Alten Orient," in *5. Internationales Colloquium der Deutschen Orient-Gesellschaft e.V.*, ed. J. Renger (in press).

conditions of drying, namely under exposure of heat, were mentioned.[18] Other terms are *urruru* "to torrefy", employed when the ingredients were to be parched, thus requiring a higher temperature, and roasted (Akk. *qalû* "to roast") which is attested only for few plants.[19]

For the extraction, simple or compound drugs were chopped, pounded, and pulverized, then dissolved in a liquid (*menstruum*). Occasionally the instrument for grinding is mentioned. Ancient Mesopotamian practitioners apparently distinguished between at least two tools depending on the nature of the ingredient. One recipe gives the instruction to grind drugs in a lead mortar (*esittu*); and to pound mineral substances, a mortar called *urṣu* was required which was probably made of stone to judge from the determinative na_4 written before the logographic spelling of the word (^{na4}NA.ZÀ.ḪI.LI).[20]

Quite a number of liquids and combinations of different liquids were used. Whether the preference for one *menstruum* over the other was dictated by what was in store, more easily available, or whether it was deliberately chosen, remains an open question. We do not know whether the choice of liquid was due to experience and observation, namely whether substances are better dissolved in oil or water.

The following liquids are attested: water, plain or in combination with the *kasû* plant,[21] milk, normal beer, strong beer, high quality beer, sesame oil, olive oil, and vinegar. Depending on the extraction method employed, a different temperature for the liquid solvent was required: cold, warm or hot.

---

18 See already Dietlinde Goltz, *Studien zur altorientalischen und griechischen Heilkunde. Therapie – Arzneibereitung – Rezeptstruktur* (Wiesbaden: Franz Steiner Verlag, 1974), 29–30. One should note here, that the drying process could take up to 14 days.

19 See Goltz, *Studien zur altorientalischen und griechischen Heilkunde*, 31.

20 We refer to the text *AMT* 82,1+ col. i: 10′, recently treated by Geller, *Renal and Rectal Disease Texts*, 90–91 (manuscript I l. 35). The line of interest which is preserved in two other duplicates (*BAM* V 430 iii′: 37′–39′ and *BAM* V 431 iii′: 40′–41′) runs as follows: "Crush the drugs in a mortar of lead, grind the 'stones' in a mortar of stone;" *šammī ina esitti abāri tušaḫḫal abnāti ina urṣi teṭên*.

21 The identification of the *kasû* plant is debated. It belonged to the basic market commodities in the second half of the 1st millenium B.C. and was used as condiment for beer, cheese, and bread. The discussion is conveniently summarized by Geller, "Review of A.L. Slotsky, The Bourse of Babylon," *Orientalistische Literaturzeitung* 95, (2000): 409–412.

2.1. *Maceration*

For maceration drugs are left in contact with the liquid for a longer period of time, usually at room temperature (59°-68°F / 15°-20°C). Needless to say, the expression "room temperature" is not stated in cuneiform prescriptions. What we find instead is the indication to keep the drugs (pounded and sieved) in the *menstruum* overnight exposed to the starry sky.

We have here two interwoven strands so illustrative for the nature of ancient Mesopotamian prescriptions: one of is materially instrumental and the other is spiritually symbolic echoing a ritual performance.[22] It is the latter aspect, the magical component that has received far more attention. The meaning and significance of exposing medications to the stars has been treated exemplarily by the late Erica Reiner in her study of *Astral Magic in Babylonia*. As she pointed out, the purpose of astral irradiation is to be understood as "to ascertain that the celestial powers make the medication efficacious; to attain this goal the medicine has to be prepared under the star's benefic influence."[23] Nevertheless, Reiner would acknowledge, following D. Goltz, that keeping drugs in a liquid solvent was also of material efficacy.[24]

It is impossible to distinguish between the motivations for depositing the drugs overnight. But in view of other methods of drug extraction that lack any divine interference, namely digestion and decoction, we may assume that the purpose of maceration was *also* due to pharmaceutical knowledge. Now, which conception was prioritized (and to which conception we give preference) – the know-how of methods for extracting drugs or magical manipulation – or to what degree the supernatural explanation had receded but was traditionally kept, and thus survived as an obsolete formula in remedies, remains an open question. It should be recalled that the majority of texts dates to the first millennium B.C. As is generally supposed, the literature of the first millennium reflects a much older tradition, coming down from the beginning of the second millennium B.C. – a phenomenon for which, in his classic presentation of ancient Mesopotamian civilization, A.L. Oppenheim coined the term

---

[22] As stated by Goltz, *Studien zur altorientalischen und griechischen Heilkunde*, 81–82. For a short reference to the method of maceration see also Schwemer, *Akkadische Rituale aus Ḫattuša*, 122, 131.

[23] Reiner, *Astral Magic*, 48.

[24] Reiner, *Astral Magic*, 48 with reference to Goltz, *Studien zur altorientalischen und griechischen Heilkunde*, 51 with fn. 300.

"stream of tradition." As he pointed out one of the characteristics of the process of standardization is maintaining "original contents against the pressures of changing concepts and attitudes."[25]

Let us turn to some of the expressions describing the procedure of maceration.[26]

By far best attested and most common is the following expression:

> "You shall keep (the macerate) overnight under the star."[27]

The second formulation specifies the star constellation corresponding to the celestial manifestation of the healing goddess Gula, demonstrating that the nocturnal exposure to the stars had more than just a practical purpose:

> "You shall keep (the macerate) overnight in front of the 'Goat-Star' (= constellation Lyra)."[28]

Alternatively, we find the phrase referring explicitly to the healing goddess:

> "You shall keep (the macerate) overnight in front of the goddess Gula."[29]

Yet another phrase appears:

> "You shall keep it overnight."[30]

It is only implicitly that these phrases state that the medication is to be kept outdoors. Very occasionally we find a reference to the usual (?) place of preparation. According to a Middle-Babylonian text written at the Hittite capital Hattuša, it was the roof which served as location:

> "On the roof you shall keep it overnight."[31]
> "You shall keep it overnight, place it on the roof."[32]

---

[25] Oppenheim, *Ancient Mesopotamia*, 18.

[26] For a full treatment of the magical aspect of irradiation see the seminal study of Reiner, *Astral Magic*, 48–59.

[27] The phrase runs in Akkadian as follows *ina kakkabi tušbât*, attested e.g. in *BAM* IV 396 i: 7′; *BAM* I 111 ii: 4′; *BAM* I 99 rev. 40; *BAM* II 168 rev. 64.

[28] See eg. *BAM* IV 396 iii: 30; *BAM* V 431 iii′: 43′: *ina pān enzi tušbât/tašakkan*.

[29] See e.g. *BAM* II 168 obv. 36; *KAR* 73 rev. 5: *ina pān gula tušbât*.

[30] *KUB* 37 no. 45 iv: 4′: *ina mu-ši-ta tu-uš-ba-a-at*.

[31] *KUB* 4 no. 48 iii: 3: *ina ú-ri ana kakkabi* [*tuš-bat*], published in transliteration and translation by Robert D. Biggs, *ŠÀ.ZI.GA. Ancient Mesopotamian Potency Incantations* (Locust Valley NY: J.J. Augustin Publisher, 1967), 55.

[32] *KUB* 4 no. 48 iii: 15 (see Biggs, *ŠÀ.ZI.GA*, 55): *ana kakkabi tuš-bat ina ú-ri ta-ša-*[*kan*].

Different verbs are attested describing the combination of drugs and their solvent, distinguishing two aspects, namely the act of blending and the act of liquefaction:

> *balālu* to mix
> "You shall mix it with oil, keep it overnight."[33]
>
> *labāku* to soak
> "You shall soak it, keep it overnight."[34]
>
> *maḫāṣu* to stir
> "You shall stir it all together and keep it overnight."[35]
>
> *nadû* to throw
> "You shall throw it into water, keep it overnight."[36]
>
> *rabāku* to moisten
> "You shall moisten it with beer, keep it overnight."[37]
>
> *ramāku* to drench
> "You shall drench it in first quality beer, keep it overnight."[38]
>
> *raṣanu* to steep
> "You shall steep it in water, keep it overnight."[39]

2.2. *Digestion*

For the procedure of digestion drugs are mixed with a *menstruum* and kept in a closed container at a higher temperature (104°-122°F / 40°-50°C). Different formulations can be found in cuneiform recipes, common to all is the enclosure in a kiln or domed oven, which allowed leavened bread to be baked.[40] It is quite likely that the remaining heat was used. Again we can observe the variation from short expressions to more detailed explanations.

Examples:

> Grind together these 25 drugs and aromatic plants (and) sieve them. Take beer of first quality, water in combination with *kasû* plant and strong

---

[33] *BAM* V 436 vi′: 11: *ina šamni tuballal ina kakkabi tuš-bat.*

[34] *BAM* VI 574 i: 23: *tu-la-bak ina kakkabi tuš-bat.*

[35] *AMT* 97,4 l. 20′: [*ištē*]*niš ta-maḫ-ḫaṣ-ma ina kakkabi tuš-bat.*

[36] *BAM* VI 579 i: 12: *ana mê tanaddi ina kakkabi tuš-bat.*

[37] *AMT* 91,5 l. 7′: *ina šikari tar-bak ina kakkabi tuš-bat.* See for the term *rabāku* also the disccussion under 4. Infusion.

[38] *AMT* 1,3 l. 9′: *ina šikari rēštî tar-muk ina kakkabi tuš-bat.*

[39] *AMT* 85,1 ii: 4: *ina mê tàr-ṣa-an ina kakkabi tuš-bat.*

[40] For a discussion of ovens used for making bread see Robert I. Curtis, *Ancient Food Technology* (Leiden / Boston / Köln: Brill, 2001), 207–208.

vinegar. Sprinkle these pulverized plants on it. Enclose it in a domed oven, remove it the next morning (and) let it cool off.[41]

Pound together these 18 drugs in equal shares, soak them in beer and vinegar, enclose it in a kiln (and) remove it the next morning.[42]

Soak these six drugs in beer, enclose it a domed oven, remove it (and) let it cool off.[43]

2.3. *Decoction*

In preparing a decoction drugs are doused in a cold *menstruum*, which is then brought to a boil. The verb used is Akk. *bašālu* which can mean both, "to boil" and "to heat".

Examples:

"You shall enclose it in a domed oven, as soon as it has boiled."[44]

Sometimes the prescriptions stress explicitly that the decoction has to be boiled such as the following recipe (note here the double meaning of Akk. *bašālu*):

"You shall heat it in a ... as soon as it has boiled."[45]

From time to time the recipient for the preparation is mentioned, a kettle made of bronze (Akk. *ruqqu*) or a bowl of earthenware (Akk. *diqāru*), but as a rule we just find the instruction to heat.

"You shall bring it to a boil in a bronze kettle (and) filter it."[46]

"You shall let it boil together with 2 l. of vinegar in a bowl (and) let it cool off."[47]

"Boil 11 drugs in first quality beer, filter it (and) let it cool off."[48]

---

41 *BAM* II 168 obv. 28–31: 25 *šammī* / *u riqqī annûti ištēniš taḫaššal tanappi šikara rēštâ mê kasê* / *u ṭābāte dannāte teleqqe itti qēmī an-nu-ti ana libbi tanaddi* / *ina tinūri tesekker ina še-rim tušellâ tukaṣṣa*; cf. also Geller, *Renal and Rectal Disease Texts*, 204–205.

42 *BAM* II 168 rev. 57–59: 18 *šammī annûti* / *mal-ma-liš ištēniš ta-ka-sim ina šikari u ṭābāti* / *tu-lab-bak ina a-tu-gi tesekker ina še-rim tušellâ-ma*; cf. also Geller, *Renal and Rectal Disease Texts*, 208–209.

43 *AMT* 47,1 + iii: 23–24: *šammī* [*annûti*] / [*ina šikari tarabbak* / *ina tinūri te-se*]*k-ker tušellâ-ma tu-kaṣ-ṣa*; cf. also Geller, *Renal and Rectal Disease Texts*, on pp. 152–155.

44 *BAM* II 122 obv. 12–13: *ina tinūri* / *tesekker ul-tu ib-taš-lu*.

45 *BAM* I 52 obv. 14: [*ina ... tu*]*baššal ki-ma ib-taš-*[*l*]*u*.

46 *BAM* II 171 obv. 16′–17′: *i-na ruqqi* / *tu-šab-šal tu-šá-ḫal*.

47 *BAM* IV 396 i: 26′–27′: 2 *qa ṭābāte ištēniš ina diqāri tu-šab-šal* / *tukaṣṣa*.

48 *BAM* I 88 rev. 23′–24′: 11 *šammī* / *ina šikari rēštî tušabšal ta-šá-ḫal tukaṣṣa*; cf. also Geller, *Renal and Rectal Disease Texts*, 170–171.

2.4. *Infusion (?)*

It should be anticipated that there is not sufficient information in recipe texts to suggest the preparation of an infusion. If we include the term here, it is to illustrate the existing lexicographic problems when dealing with medical cuneiform texts.

If the liquid solvent is boiling and then poured over the drugs, we speak of an infusion. According to the two main dictionaries of the Akkadian language, the verb *rabāku* was used to denote the action of "to decoct, to make an infusion" (*CAD* R 8a) and "einen Absud herstellen" (*AHw* 933b). It was Benno Landsberger who established this meaning in one of his volumes of Materialien zum sumerischen Lexikon (MSL), which then entered both dictionaries.[49] In his commentary he rejects an earlier suggestion proposed by Friedrich Küchler who, on etymological grounds, favoured a translation "to mix, to stir."[50] In 1974 Dietlinde Goltz discussed the verb anew and argued on the basis of the pharmaceutical context of the recipes that a meaning "to stir" is rather preferable.[51] Earlier, René Labat had put forward another translation understanding the verb as "to mix, to moisten."[52] Though we agree with the argumentation of Goltz that the consistency of the required medication is rather a mash than a liquid since the preparation of a poultice is recommended, we prefer to follow Labat's translation "to moisten."

Occasionally, the use of a boiling liquid, namely of hot or boiling water in combination with *kasû* plant or beer is attested. The prescriptions in question seem to point to the preparation of cataplasms or poultices, so that the hot liquid was possibly only employed in order to allow the drugs to swell up rather than to produce an infusion.

3. *Forms of Medication*

A number of forms of medication were used by ancient Mesopotamian practitioners such as potions, foods, salves, bandages, poultices, powders,

---

[49] *Die Serie* Ur-e-a = *nâqu*, MSL 2 (Roma: Pontificium Institutum Biblicum, 1951), 110.

[50] F. Küchler, *Beiträge zur Kenntnis der assyrisch-babylonischen assyrisch Medizin*, Assyrische Bibliothek 18 (Leipzig: Hinrichs, 1904), 103.

[51] Goltz, *Studien zur altorientalischen und griechischen Heilkunde*, 47.

[52] R. Labat, "Le premier chapitre d'un précis médical assyrien," *Revue d'Assyriologie* 53 (1959): 1–18, on p. 5 line 15.

pills, pessaries, tampons, enemas, suppositories, drops, lotions, insufflations of drugs, inhalations and fumigations. An overview has been provided by Goltz who briefly discussed forms of medication as well as some of the diseases treated.[53] Her study is hitherto the only structural approach to cuneiform prescriptions. Although in many respects it is still valid, a revision and enlargement is a desideratum, due to the increasing number of publications of medical texts. In what follows we shall examine and re-evaluate two forms of medication, namely the administration of enemas and the preparation of suppositories. The following study has profited from the recent translation of recipe texts dealing with renal and anal diseases published by Markham J. Geller.[54]

3.1. *Enema*

The Akkadian verb describing the administration of an enema is *šapāku* "to pour." The expression in full runs as follows: *ana šuburrī*(DÚR)-*šú tašappak*(DUB-*ak*), "you shall pour / inject it into his anus." The enema itself is called in Akkadian *maṣraḫu* "lotion, liquid (for inserting)" derived from the verb *raḫāṣu* "to wash, to bathe" as discussed already by Goltz.[55]

Though it is rare, additional information about the instruments for applying enemas can be found. We know of two tools for applying enemas: the first is mentioned in a small fragmentary text unearthed at the ancient city of Assur; it is a tool in the shape of a flute made of reed and wrapped in cloth, called in Akkadian *embūbu*.[56] The second instrument is attested not only in context of human medicine but also in a veterinary prescription. According to one of the few veterinary recipes for curing a horse, an enema administered through a leather hose is called *mašqītu*.[57] The other attestation comes from a prescription belonging to

---

[53] Goltz, *Studien zur altorientalischen und griechischen Heilkunde*, 60–86.

[54] Geller, *Renal and Rectal Disease Texts, Die babylonisch-assyrische Medizin* VII; cf. the author's review article of the text edition "Babylonisch-assyrische Medizin in Texten und Untersuchungen: Erkrankungen des uro-genitalen Traktes, des Enddarmes und des Anus," *Wiener Zeitschrift für die Kunde des Morgenlandes* 98 (2008): 295–346.

[55] Goltz, *Studien zur altorientalischen und griechischen Heilkunde*, 79.

[56] The term is attested in *BAM* I 104 obv. 20 *embūbu*; see for the line Geller, *Renal and Rectal Disease Texts*, 174–175. The dictionaries of the Akkadian language do not list a meaning "tube," the translations provided according to the context are "flute" and "windpipe;" see *CAD* E, 137b and *AHw*, 180b.

[57] See *CAD* M/1, 384a.

human medicine and makes reference to the same tool, a leather hose: "You shall fill it (= the lotion) in a leather hose (and) inject it into his anus."[58]

As can be observed, prescriptions for the medication of enemas feature two different characteristics: often exact amounts are provided in contrast to the rather common practice of dropping measurements, and the number of drugs employed can go up to nearly 100.[59] The preparation of drugs includes maceration, digestion and decoction. The liquid is then mixed with carriers such as olive or sesame oil and mixtures of syrup and oil.[60]

Among other effects, enemas were applied because of their irrigating effect thus removing all harmful waste products of the human body, which may symbolically stand for the purification and expulsion of diseases and demons.[61] We hardly dispose of exact information about the degree to which ancient Mesopotamians were conscious about body functions. What we know is how they imagined the digestive tract. According to an incantation, the intestines resembled canals supervised by an inspector – a metaphor that reflects strikingly well the environmental reality of southern Mesopotamia. The incantation runs as follows: "Whom should I send to the canal inspector of your innards? May they bring with them silver spates and golden shovels! May they open the canals, may they open the ditches! May his excrements get way, may it come out! May the storm in his belly come out!"[62]

Recipe texts describe the effect of an enema with two verbs: *nasāḫu* "to tear out, to expel" and *šaḫāṭu* "to rinse, to clean."[63] Both terms seem to allude again to the two elements of ancient Mesopotamian medicine, magical manipulation and physical effect.

---

58 *BAM* VI 574 ii: 20: *ana* [kuš]*maš-qí-ti te-si-ip ana šuburrī-šú tašappak.*

59 As for e.g. stated in *BAM* V 430 iii′: 35′ (94 drugs); note that the duplicate *AMT* 82,1+ i: 34 (for which see Geller, *Renal and Rectal Disease Texts*, 90 l. 34) preserves the number 90+[ ].

60 See e.g. for the mixture of syrup and oil the text *AMT* 56,1 rev. 3′ (cf. Geller, *Renal and Rectal Disease Texts*, 196–197); for oil see e.g. *BAM* I 52 obv. 7.

61 As put forward by Goltz, *Studien zur altorientalischen und griechischen Heilkunde*, 79, 81–82.

62 See for the edition of the incantation Walter Farber, "*Mannam lupšur ana Enkidu*: Some Thoughts About an Old Motif," *Journal of Near Eastern Studies* 49 (1990): 219–321, p. 319–320.

63 See for example the prescription of an enema "in order to expel the disease caused by the 'hand of the the oath'" (*STT* I 97 ii: 6′: [*ana*] *qāt māmīti nasā*[*ḫi*]). Other enemas serve "to tear out fever" see *BAM* VI 579 i: 51 *ana ummi libbi nasāḫi*, or "to tear out the fever of the head" see BM 47943 obv. 27 *ana ummi qaqqadi nasāḫi*. For the usage of the

Enemas were prescribed for diseases of the digestive tract, covering afflictions of the small and large intestines and the rectum, diseases of the upper alimentary canal, afflictions of the kidneys and the pelvic area, and also for cases of fever and jaundice. As for the therapeutic effect, one could perhaps cautiously apply the modern usages: cleansing enemas for flushing out the colon, retention enemas for introducing medication into the rectum, and carminative enemas for distending the rectum and releasing gas.

A note on the diseases treated is in order here. We do not venture to identify ancient diseases on the basis of the cuneiform recipes because we consider that neither the nature of the cuneiform sources nor the information they provide nor the ancient Mesopotamian concept of disease allow a verification of possible identifications.[64] It should further be mentioned that our proper understanding of anatomical expressions in Akkadian is seriously hampered by polysemy. A good example is the term *libbu*, which refers depending on the context to the heart, the belly, the stomach, the intestines, the innards, the body or the "feelings".

In what follows we give preference to the form of medication, thus giving first examples for mono-phase treatments recommending exclusively the application of an enema, then multiphase cures which prescribe in addition potions, suppositories, fumigations, etc.

a. *Mono-Phase Treatments*

Dried faeces – Cleansing enema

> If a man's faeces are dried in his intestines, he is sick with the disease called *zizibēnu* – in order to heal him: let 0,33 l. of glasswort, 0,3 l. of strong wine

verb *šaḫāṭu* see e.g. *BAM* II 168 rev. 62 "in order to rinse out the fever of his belly" *ummi libbī-*[*šú*] *šá-ḫa-ṭi* (see Geller, *Renal and Rectal Disease Texts*, 208–209).

[64] One should refer here to the discussion of the interpretative problems posed by the method of retrospective diagnosis by Karl-Heinz Leven; see e.g. his contributions "Krankheiten – historische Deutung versus retrospektive Diagnose," in *Medizingeschichte: Aufgaben, Probleme, Perspektiven*, eds. Norbert Paul / Thomas Schlich, (Frankfurt am Main/New York: Campus Fachbuch, 1998), 153–185, and "Retrospective Diagnosis and Ancient Medical History," in *Magic and Rationality in Ancient Near Eastern and Graeco-Roman Medicine*, eds. Manfred Horstmanshoff / Marten Stol, (Leiden/Boston: Brill, 2004), 369–386. Recently, Scurlock and Andersen have published a massive on the diagnosis of Akkadian diseases, *Diagnoses in Assyrian and Babylonian Medicine*. The work, as valuable as it may seem, presses the Ancient Mesopotamian concept of disease into our modern scheme. For a more detailed criticism of the book, see the present author's contribution "Diagnose im Alten Mesopotamien" forthcoming in *Orientalistische Literaturzeitung*.

vinegar, 41,65 g of salt (and) 41,65 g of mint[65] boil in high quality beer, add oil to it, inject it into his rectum.[66]

Expelling flatus – Carminative enema

Aromatic *kukrû* plant, juniper, aromatic *suādu* plant, 'bitter plant', 'lung (plant)', glasswort, *nuḫurtu* plant, *urnû* plant, *kasû* plant, salt, sweet reed, date. 12 drugs, dosage for releasing flatus, inject it into his rectum and he shall recover.[67]

Flatus, abdominal distension, haemorrhoids[68] – Carminative enema

If a man is sick with stricture of the bladder: 16,66 g 'bitter plant', 16,66 g of resin of the aromatic *baluḫḫu* plant, water in combination with 'lung (plant)', with *nuḫurtu* plant, with salt (and) with all other kinds of aromata. Take of each type of water 500 ml, crush (all ingredients) together, let it boil, sieve it, let it cool off, mix it with 500 ml of oil. Crush 0,35 g of mandrake, sprinkle it over (the liquid). Divide the liquid into three parts and inject it once, twice, thrice into his rectum. His flatulence will be expelled (literally: the accumulation of his intestines will be relieved), in case of haemorrhoids of the *uršu* type they will be destroyed, in case of haemorrhoids of the *umṣatu* type they will be plucked off, the affliction will be appeased, his rectum will be distended. This is an enema for releasing (evil machinations caused by) curse and for all kinds of diseases.[69]

Flatus, stinging pain in the body, feeling of paralysis, bad smell, distorted features – Carminative enema

If flatus lets a man's intestines quiver (and) he suffers from flatulence, his body, his legs, his breast and his shoulders hurt him constantly, all his flesh

---

65 For the more recent discussion of the identification of *nīnû* with mint see James V. Kinnier Wilson, "The Assyrian Pharmaceutical Series URU.AN.NA," *Journal of Near Eastern Studies* 64 (2005): 45–51, on pp. 50–51.

66 *AMT* 40,4+ rev. 1–5: [*šumma amēlu*] *šit-ta-šú ina lìb-bi-šú i-ta-nab-bal* / [*amēlu š*]*û zi-zi-*⟨*be*⟩*-na maruṣ ana bulluṭī-šú* 1/3 *qa uḫūla qarnāna* / 1/3 *qa mê karāni danni* 5 *šiqil ṭa-ab-ti* / 5 *šiqil nīnâ ina šikari rēštî tušabšal šamna* / *ana pāni tanaddi ana šuburrī-šú tušappak*; see also Geller, *Renal and Rectal Disease Texts*, 184–185 (rev. ll. 14′–18′).

67 *BAM* I 54 obv. 13–15: *kukru burāšu suādu murru ḫašû uḫūlu qarnānu nuḫurtu* / [ú]*úr-ni-e kasû tābṭu qānu ṭābu suluppu* 12 *šammī* [*annûti*] / [*taḫ-ḫ*]*i-it-ti šāra parāsi ana šuburrī-šú tušappak* [*iballuṭ*].

68 What is here translated with haemorrhoids corresponds in Akkadian to two terms designating abnormal appearances of the skin.

69 *BAM* II 168 rev. 45–53: *šumma amēlu ḫi-niq-ti ellabuḫḫi maruṣ* 2 *šiqil murra* 2 *šiqil ḫīl baluḫḫi* / *mê ḫašê mê nuḫurti mê ṭābti mê riqqê kalî-šú-nu* / *mê šú-nu-ti* 1/2 *qa ištēnâ teleqqe ištēniš taḫaššal tušabšal* / *ta-šá-ḫal tukaṣṣa* 1/2 *šamna ittī-šú-nu tuballal* 7 *uṭṭet šammi balāṭi* / *tazâk ana libbi tanaddi mê ana šalāšī-šú ta-za-az-ma* / *ištēn-šú šinī-šú šalāšī-šú ana šuburrī-šú tašappak e-sil-ti libbī-šú ušeššer* / *šum-ma ur-še iḫtepû šum-ma um-ṣa-a-tú uq-ṭa-ta-pa* / *simmu up-ta-šaḫ šuburra-šú ur-tap-pa-áš mar-ḫa-ṣu an-nu-u* / *ša namerimburrudê murṣi kalîšu*; cf. also Geller, *Renal and Rectal Disease Texts*, 206–207.

has become paralyzed and causes him sharp pain, his flesh is wasting away, bad smell surrounds him, his complexion is distorted, he is hot all day long, in order to heal him: aromatic *kukrû* plant, juniper, *atā'išu* plant, 'lung (plant)', *saḫlû* plant, *kasû* plant, red salt, *urnû* plant, twig of tamarisk. Crush these nine drugs together, moisten it with good wine and high quality beer, keep it during the night under the stars, boil it the next morning, filter it, let it cool off, crush together 0,35 g of the seed of the *irrû* colocynth (and) 0,35 g of *anzaḫḫu* mineral, pound it all together, let him drink it before sunrise, induce him to vomit with a feather, if he is not in good health, inject it into his rectum, he shall recover.[70]

"Fever of the innards" – Cleansing enema (?)[71]

In order to tear out fever of the innards: 'bitter plant', aromatic *šumuttu* plant, sweet reed, 'lung (plant)', – broken –, *nuḫurtu* plant, date, aromatic *kukru* plant. Crush these seven drugs together, sieve it, soak it in beer, enclose it in a domed oven, remove it and filter it. Let it cool off. Add lumps of malt to it, let it deposit, add water in combination with *kasû* plant to it. Inject this into his rectum and he shall recover.[72]

"Hand of the spirit of the dead", abdominal disease *durgiqqû*, kidneys – Retention enema

Add ..., soak aromatic *ṭiru* plant, as soon as you have let it soaked add to it cedar resin (and) filtered oil which you have emulsified. Mix these drugs together with it (the emulsion), filter it through a cloth, inject it into his rectum and he shall recover. This is a lotion (enema) for (afflictions caused by) the 'Hand of the spirit of the dead', the abdominal *durgiqqû* disease and to relax the kidneys. Begin (the treatment) and he shall recover.[73]

---

[70] *BAM* VI 575 iii: 30–36: *šumma amēlu šāru ina libbī-šú uš-tar-'a-ab [i-li-ḫi-ib] u zumur-šú šēpīšu irassu u naglabū-šú / ītanakkalū-šú šīrū-šú ú-šam-ma-[mu-šú u izzanaq-qatū]-šú šīrū-šú ma-ṭu-u ni-ip-še mali zīmū-šú i-ta-na-nu-ú / ītenemmem ina kal u_4-me ú-gil-šu [ana bulluṭī-šú kukru] burāšu atā'išu ḫašû saḫ-lí-e kasû / tābaṭ a-ma-nim* ${}^{\acute{u}}$*úr-ni-e ār b[i-ni 9 šam]mī annûti ištēniš tazâk ina karāni ṭābi u šikari rēštê ta-ra-sa-an / ina mūši ana pān kakkabi tuš-bat ina šēri [tušabšal] ta-šá-ḫal tukaṣṣa 7 uṭṭāt ḫabbur irrê / 7 uṭṭāt anzaḫḫa ištēniš tazâk iš[tēniš taḫa]ššal la-am šamaš na-pa-ḫi tušaqqī-šú / ina agappi tu-šap-ra-šú šum*$_4$*-ma ṭūba lā īmur ana šuburrī-šú tašappak iballuṭ.*

[71] It is not clear how the following recipe works. On the basis of the term "to expel, tear out" preference has been given to the idea of cleansing the body from harmful waste.

[72] *BAM* VI 579 i: 51–54: *ana ummi libbi nasāḫi murru suādu qānu ṭābu ḫašû / ḫe-pí nuḫurtu suluppu kukru 7 šammī an-nu-ti ištēniš taḫaššal tanappi / ina šikari tar-muk ina tinūri tesekker* ⸢*tušellâ-ma*⸣ *ta-šá-ḫal tukaṣṣa šibirti buqli ana libbi tanaddi tašakkan / ina pa-ni mê kasê tan[add]i an-na-a ana šuburrī-šú [tašapp]ak-ma iballuṭ.*

[73] *BAM* III 222 obv. 1–9: [*ta*]*naddi ṭira ina lìb-bi / tu-rab-ba ki-ma tur-tab-bi / dām erēni šamna ḫal-ṣa šá tu-sa-me-ḫu / ina muḫḫi a-ḫa-meš tanaddī-šú-nu-ti / šammī an-nu-ti ana libbi a-ḫa-meš tu-sa-maḫ / ina ṣubāti ta-šá-ḫal ina šuburrī-šú tašappak-ma iballuṭ / an-nu-ú mar-ḫaṣ ša qāt eṭemmi / durguqqî u kalīti lu-ub-bi-ki / tušarrâ-ma iballuṭ.*

Jaundice – Retention enema

If a man has been seized, be it that he is sick of gall, be it the 'catcher-demon' who causes jaundice, or be it that he is sick of jaundice – in order to heal him: aromatic *kukru* plant, juniper, aromatic *ballukku* plant, aromatic *suādu* plant, sweet reed, *urnû* plant, *atā'išu* plant, 'fox-wine', *karšu* plant, *bū'šānu* plant, *tarmuš* plant, 'It-stood-against-1000', 'It-stood-against-20', *irrû* colocynth. Weigh equal amounts of these 14 drugs, let it boil in high quality beer, keep it under the stars, in the morning sieve it, add oil (and) syrup to it, inject it into his rectum.[74]

Intestinal parasites – Retention enema

If a man's intestines have caught the intestinal parasites *urbatu*, *quqānu* (or) *pilû*, crush 0,7 g of the peel of the plant called 'It-stood-against-1000', pound it with pressed oil, inject it into his rectum and he shall recover.[75]

Stiff hips – Retention enema

In order to relax stiff hips: bring malt, linseed, aromatic *suādu* plant, aromatic *ballukku* plant, sweet reed, 'bitter plant' (and) *sikkatu* plant to a boil in oil and beer, inject it into his rectum.[76]

b. *Multiphase Treatments*

Dry throat, shortness of breath, vomiting gall – Cleansing enema (?)

If a man's breast/bronchia is/are afflicted and his throat is as if it would be obstructed with dry dusty stuff, when he talks he is constantly short of breath and continually vomits gall, this man suffers from 'property of his belly,' in order to heal him: let him drink on an empty stomach 'dog's tongue plant' in beer. Wash him constantly with water in combination with *kasû* plant, inject water in combination with chaste berry into his rectum. He sucks up through a tube pea flour (and) *urnû* plant with his mouth. You mix together aromatic *ṭiru* plant, pith of dates, juniper (and) aromatic *kukru* plant, apply it on leather, bandage him.[77]

---

[74] *BAM* II 188 1–10: *šumma amēlu iṣbassu lu martu lu aḫ-ḫa-zu / lu a-mur-ri-qa-nu maruṣ ana bulluṭī-šú / kukru burāšu ballukku / suādu qānu ṭābu* ^{ú}*úr-nu-u / atā'išu karān šēlebi* ^{ú}*kar-šú / bū'šānu* ^{giš}*tar-muš*$_8$ ^{giš}*imḫur-lim* ^{giš}*imḫur-ešrā /* ^{ú}*ir-ru-u* 14 *šammī an-nu-ti / mal-ma-liš tašaqqal ina šikari rēštî tušabšal / ina kakkabi tuš-bat ina še-rim ta-šá-ḫal / šamna dišpa ana pāni tanaddi ana šuburrī-šú tašappak.*

[75] *BAM* II 159 ii: 43–45: *šumma amēlu libba-šú ur-ba-tu qu-qa-nu-u pi-lu-u / ṣabit* 14 *uṭṭet qilip* ^{ú}*imḫur-lim tazâk ina šamni ḫal-ṣi / taḫaššal ana šuburrī-šú tašappak-ma iballuṭ.*

[76] *AMT* 56,1 rev.5′–6′: [*ana qablī*] *áš-ṭa-a-te lu-ub-bu-ka šibirti buqli zēr kitê suāda / ballukka qanâ ṭāba murra sik-ka-ti ina šamni u šikari tušabšal ana šuburri tašappak*; cf. also Geller, *Renal and Rectal Disease Texts*, 196–197.

[77] *BAM* VI 575 iii: 55–58: *šumma amēlu irassu marṣat-ma kīma ši-ne-e-ti epera irtanašši ina da-ba-bi-šú ik-ka-šú ik-ta-ner-ru / ù marta ip-te-nar-ru amēlu šû bi-šit libbi*

Fatigue, unability to defecate – Cleansing enema

If fatigue has caught a man and he cannot defecate, boil high quality beer in a bronze bowl, add salt to it, inject it into his rectum. Wrap your finger into (a piece of) linen, coat it with salt, apply it to his rectum, place into his anus the 'Pubic-hair-of-an-old-woman [...].[78]

Abdominal distension – Carminative enema

If a man's intestines are inflamed (and) bloated, flatus churns his belly (and) he suffers from flatulence, apply pith of the *irrû* colocynth into his anus, crush garlic (and) cumin, let him constantly drink it with beer, during two days inject each day half a litre of oil into his rectum, he shall recover.[79]

Piercing pain – Retention enema

For poultice in case of piercing pain be it the right side, be it the left side: Crush separately date, ... of malt, *saḫimtu* plant, aromatic *ballukku* plant, seed of *aktam* plant (and) dry mass (for preparing) good beer, mix it all together with oil, boil it, apply it on a piece of leather, make a bandage. As soon as you have taken it off, wash him constantly with water in combination with chaste berry. (Enumeration of drugs) – 35 drugs. Boil up the lotion with beer, inject it into his rectum.[80]

---

maruṣ ana bulluṭī-šú lišān kalbi ina šikari lā pa-tan tušaqqī-šú / ina mê kasê irtanaḫḫaṣ mê šunê ana šuburrī-šú tašappak qēm kakkî [giš]*ùr-ne-e ina takkussi ina pî-šú išaddad / ṭira lipi suluppi burāša kukra ištēniš tuballal ina maški teṭerri taṣammid.*

[78] *BAM* VI 575 iii: 47–48: *šumma amēlu an-šú-tum iṣ-bat-su-ma la ú-šar-da šikara rēštâ ina tamgussi tušabšal ṭābta ana libbi tanaddi ana šuburrī-[šú tašappak-ma] / ubānka ṣubat kitê talammi ṭābta ta-ṣap-pu šuburra-šú ta-kar šārat ūri šībti ina qabal pî-šú tašakkan.* In all likelihood, the "pubic hair of an old woman" is rather the descriptive name of a plant than the actual hair. It was Köcher who studied in detail the phenomenon of descriptive and secret names of plants, see his "Ein Text medizinischen Inhalts aus dem neubabylonischen Grab 405," on p. 211 sub 5′. 8′. A list of these "hidden names" is preserved in the third chapter of the pharmaceutical handbook Uruanna:*maštakal*. Recently, Kinnier Wilson in his contribution "The Assyrian Pharmaceutical Series URU.AN.NA," *Journal of Near Eastern Studies* 64 (2005) 45–51, on pp. 48–49, has drawn attention to the classification "hidden" or "secret" of some of the plant names. As he discusses, some designations seem to have been rather riddles, whereas others were popular plant names.

[79] *BAM* VI 575 ii: 20–21: *šumma amēlu libbū-šú ittanappaḫū it-te-ni-bi-ṭu šāru ina libbī-šú issanaḫḫur i-le-bu lipi irrê ana šuburrī-šú tašakkan / šūma* [ú]*zi-ba-a tazâk ina šikari taltanaqqi 2 ūmī 1/2 qa* ta.àm *šamna ana šuburrī-šú tašappak i[balluṭ].*

[80] *BAM* I 3 iv: 35–38, 44–45: *ana na-aṣ-mad di-ik-ši lu šá 15 lu [šá] 150 suluppa tap-pi-iṣ buqli / sa-ḫi-in-du ballukka zēr* [ú]*ak-tam billata damqata a-ḫi-e tazâk / ina šamni ištēniš tuballal ina išāti tušabšal ina maški teṭerri taṣammid kīma ta-[ap-ṭa-a]ṭ-ru / ina mê šunê irtanaḫḫassu /* (ll. 38–44 enumeration of drugs) / 35 *šammī / mar-ḫaṣ ina šikari tušabšal ana šuburrī-šú tašappak.* For the restoration see the partial duplicate *AMT* 96,1 obv. 1–7.

3.2. *Suppository*

Ancient Mesopotamian practitioners distinguished between three sizes of suppositories, namely acorn size (Akkadian *allānu* "acorn"), finger size (*ubānu* "finger"), and the size of a pill (expressed with the verb *kapātu* "to roll [into a pill]").

The basic substance or carrier for suppositories and also for salves is suet extracted from the adipose tissue of the kidneys and loins of slaughtered animals. More information in the texts about the process of melting out the suet is not provided. Whereas most remedies mention suet without further classification, some do indicate the origin, namely "beef suet" or "mutton suet".[81] The terms used in Akkadian are *lipû* for suet, *lipi alpi* "beef suet" and *lipi kalīt immeri* "suet of the kidney of mutton". In addition we find combinations of different kinds of suet or mixtures of suet and wax, suet, wax and resin of the aromatic *baluḫḫu* plant, or suet and date skin.[82] One recipe coming from Ashurbanipal's palace library at Nineveh prescribes the use of cedar oil and lion suet – an ingredient that might at first sight sound astonishing.[83]

It is interesting to note that when wax was being used the carrier mass had to be heated. Although the instruction is not always attested, the warming up becomes evident if we consider the melting point of wax (bee wax) which is between 62° and 65°C (144°-149°F) and which requires a higher temperature to melt in contrast to beef suet, with 40°-43°C (104°-109°F), or mutton suet, with ca. 41°C (106°F), both becoming soft when being hand-hot. Mutton suet is of white colour, harder in consistency and rough, in contrast to beef suet, which is yellow, soft and smooth. Mutton suet is less durable than beef suet, since it quickly becomes rancid once exposed to air.

For suppositories the ingredients had to be crushed and pounded very fine before being added to the carrier. Usually, the recipes do not specify whether the medicinal plants were to be dried first or used fresh. Important additional information comes here from one of the pharmaceutical compendia, namely the plant description text "About the appearance of the medicinal plant" (Akkadian *šammu šikinšu*).[84] As far as

[81] Cf. also Geller, *Renal and Rectal Disease Texts*, 4 "oils."

[82] See Geller, *Renal and Rectal Disease Texts*, 4.

[83] See for the text passage Geller, *Renal and Rectal Disease Texts*, 150–151 (ii: 3). One should note that "Lion fat" is attested as a descriptive plant name.

[84] A study and edition of this handbook is being prepared by the present author.

the handbook is preserved, some plants are qualified as being especially "good for the rectum." The plants mentioned are simple drugs like the "bitter plant" (*murru*) which is to be used in "its green / fresh state" (*arqūssu*), or the herbs "spittle-from-the-ground" (*gišût qaqqari*) and the *irrû* colocynth which both had to be dried, crushed and mixed with oil before being shaped into a "finger" suppository.[85]

Among the diseases and afflictions treated with suppositories we find a severe abdominal and rectal disease called in Akkadian *durgiqqû*. The symptoms range from pains in the extremities and constipation to defecating blood.[86] Other ailments include flatulence, discharging blood, haemorrhoids, and afflictions of the rectum.

In what follows we quote some examples for the use of suppositories constituting mono-phase treatments.

Having suffered from the abdominal *durgiqqû* disease in youth

> If a man suffers too early for his age from pains in his hip, his shins cause him piercing pain, his thighs are exhausted, his genitals feel cold, this man has suffered ⟨from the *durgiqqû* disease⟩ in his youth. [In order to heal him]: mint, *atā'išu* plant, *saḫlû* plant, potash, 'white drug',[87] *nuḫurtu* plant, *gabû* mineral, aromatic *kukru* plant, juniper, 'bitter plant', resin of the

[85] For the "bitter plant" see *KADP* 33 obv. 10–11: *šammu šû murru šum*[*šu*] / *ana šuburri damiq arqūssu ana šuburrī-šu tašakkan-ma iballuṭ*, "This plant is called 'bitter plant'. It is good for the rectum. When it is green / fresh you apply it to his rectum and he shall recover." The plant *murru* is identified with myrrh (*Balsamodendron myrrha* Nees, see Campbell Thompson, *A Dictionary*, 339–340), which has been challenged by W. Farber, "Myrrhe. B. Philologisch," *Reallexikon der Assyriologie* 8 (1993–1997): 536–537. For the plant 'spittle-from-the-ground' see *KADP* 33 rev. 8′–9′: *šammu šû* ${}^{\text{ú}}$*gi-šu-ut qaqqari šum-šú* / *ana šuburri damiq tubbal tazâk itti šamni tuballal ubāna teppuš ana šuburrī -šú tašakkan-ma iballuṭ*, "This plant is called 'spittle-from-the-ground'. It is good for the rectum. Dry it, pound it, mix it with oil, form a 'finger' suppository, introduce it into his rectum and he shall recover." For the *irrû* colocynth see *STT* I 93 rev. 67′: *šammu šû irrû* [*šumšu*] *ana šuburri es-*[*l*]*i damiq tubbal tazâk itti šamni tuballal ana šuburrī-šú tašakkan-*⌈*ma*⌉ [*iballuṭ*], "This plant is called *irrû* colocynth. It is good for constipated rectum. Dry it, pound it, mix it with oil, apply it to his rectum and he shall recover."

[86] Pains in the hips, knees and genitals are stated in the text *AMT* 43,1+ i: 1–2 (and duplicates), "If a man too young for his age has constantly pains in his hips, his knees cause him piercing pain, his genitals are cold"; see Geller, *Renal and Rectal Disease Texts*, pp. 136–137. Constipation is mentioned in *BAM* I 95 obv. 21 for which see Geller, *Renal and Rectal Disease Texts*, pp. 130–131. For the symptom of blood see the same text *BAM* I 95 rev. 27–28 (Geller, *Renal and Rectal Disease Texts*, on pp. 132–133).

[87] We translate the Akkadian term (or its logographic representation) literally. The "white drug" (*šammu peṣû*) is explained as the sap of the poplar according to the medical text *AMT* 40,5 iv: 23′: *šammu peṣû šá ḫīl ṣarbati* (see for the text also Geller, *Renal and Rectal Diseases*, 146–147).

aromatic *abukattu* plant (and) salt. Crush these 12 drugs separately, sieve it, mix it with mutton suet, bee wax and resin of the aromatic *baluḫḫu* plant, heat it up, form an 'acorn' suppository, introduce it into his rectum and he shall recover.[88]

To relieve from flatulence

(Enumeration of drugs). Crush these 15 drugs together, sieve it, mix it with suet and skin of dates, grind it in a mortar. Sprinkle oil on it. Form an 'acorn' suppository, dampen with ghee, introduce it into his rectum, and the pent-up flatus shall come out. Proven recipe.[89]

To expel flatus

Dates from the land of Dilmun, glasswort, mutton suet, aromatic *kukru* plant, juniper, aromatic *ṣumlalû* plant, resin of the aromatic *baluḫḫu* plant, resin of the *abukkatu* plant. 8 ingredients. 'Acorn'-suppository for expelling flatus. Introduce it into his rectum. Proven recipe.[90]

Discharging blood through the anus

If a man discharges blood through his anus, he suffers from an affliction of the inside of his rectum. In order to heal him: aromatic *kukru* plant, glasswort, *atā'išu* plant, mint, *saḫlû* plant, resin of the aromatic *baluḫḫu* plant. Crush these 7 ingredients together, mix it with mutton suet, form an 'acorn' suppository, introduce it into his anus and he shall recover.[91]

Inflammation of the anus, haemorrhoids

If a man's anus (literally: the mouth of his rectum) is constantly inflamed (and) hardened, the inside (of the rectum) is afflicted, there are haemorrhoids of the *umṣatu* type. Crush resin of the aromatic plant *abukattu*, seed

---

[88] *AMT* 43,1+ i: 1–2, 7–10: *šumma amēlu ina la si-ma-ni-šú qabal-šú ītanakkal-šú kim-ṣa-a-*[*šú i-za-qa*]*ta-šú* / *bur-ka-šú i-ka-ṣa-a-šú amēlu šû ina meṣ-ḫi-ru-ti-šú* ⟨*durgiqqâ*⟩ *maruṣ* / (ll. 7–10) [*ana bulluṭī-šú*] *nīnâ atā'iša saḫ-lí-e uḫūla qarnāna qa-la-te šamma peṣâ* / *nuḫurta* [na4]*ga-bi-i kukra burāša murra ḫīl a-bu-ka-tim* / *ṭābta* 12 *šammī an-nu-ti a-ḫi-en-na taḫaššal* [*tanappi*] *ina lipê iškūri* / *ḫīl baluḫḫi tušabšal tuballal allāna teppuš ana* [*šuburrī-šú*] *tašakkan-ma ina-eš*; cf. also Geller, *Renal and Rectal Disease Texts*, 136–137.

[89] *BAM* II 152 iii: 4–7: 15 *šammī annûti ištēniš taḫaššal tanappi* / *ina lipê u qí-lip suluppi tuballal tutār-ma ina esitti taḫaššal šamna iltanappat alla-nu teppuš ḫimēta tasallaḫ ana šuburrī-šú tašakkan-ma šāru es-lu uṣṣâ bul-ṭu lat-ku.*

[90] *BAM* II 168 rev. 78–81 (and duplicates): *suluppa tilmunâ uḫūla qarnāna lipi kalīt immeri* / *kukra burāša ṣumlalâ ḫīl baluḫḫi* / *ḫīl abukkati* 8 *šammū* / *alla-nu šāra parāsi ana šuburrī-šú tašakkan bul-ṭu lat-*[*ku*]; cf. also Geller, *Renal and Rectal Disease Texts*, 128–129.

[91] *BAM* I 95 rev. 29–30 (and duplicates): *šumma amēlu dāma ina šuburrī-šú ú-tab-ba-ka amēlu šû qer-bé-ni šuburri maruṣ ana* [*bulluṭī*]*-šú kukra burāša uḫūla qarnāna atā'iša nīnâ* / *saḫ-lí-e ḫīl baluḫḫi* 7 *šammī an-nu-ti ištēniš tazâk ina lipi kalīt immeri tuballal alla-nu teppuš ana šuburrī-šú tašakkan-ma iballuṭ*; cf. also Geller, *Renal and Rectal Disease Texts*, 132–133.

> of the *aktam* plant, the plant with the descriptive name 'excrement of a dog', root of male mandrake, mint, garlic consisting of one clove, 'cobweb' plant, fruit of the *kalbānu* plant, mix it with suet, form a 'finger' suppository, introduce it into his rectum.[92]

Stricture of the anus through haemorrhoids

> If a man's anus is constricted and his anus is covered with haemorrhoids of the *umṣatu* and the *urše* type, in order to heal him: mix together in equal quantities mint, juniper, aromatic *kanaktu* plant, 'plant of life', together with suet and resin of the aromatic *baluḫḫu* plant, form a 'finger' suppository, introduce it into his rectum and he shall recover.[93]

A rectal disease

> If a man's anus is afflicted and his rectum is pent-up, crush bat guano (and) root of male mandrake, mix it, roll it together into a pill, introduce it into his rectum and he shall recover.[94]

4. *Concluding Remarks*

Cuneiform recipes exhibit a variety of techniques employed for the preparation of medicaments. They belong in the words of A. Leo Oppenheim to a group of texts which contain "procedural instructions" and fall "into the category of what we consider today the exact sciences."[95] This group includes instructions for the manufacturing of glass and perfumes, as well as recipes for the production of beer.

As far as the study of medical texts is concerned and considering the state of publication of the extant material, we are still far away from presenting a precise description of all aspects of ancient Mesopotamian medical know-how. In this regard the study presented here about drug extraction methods and two forms of medication is an initial analysis. As could be observed in some prescriptions, magical and technical

[92] *BAM* I 104 obv. 42–44 (and duplicates): [*šumma amēlu pî šuburrī*]-*šú ittanappaḫ ú-na-paq qer-bé-nu maruṣ um-ṣa-tum ḫīl* / [*a-ku-ka*]-*tum zēr* ᵘ*ak-tam zê kalbi išid pillî zikari nīnâ tu*-[*ra*] / [*penzer inib*] *kalbāni tazâk ina lipê tuballal ubāna teppuš ina šuburrī-šú tašakkan*; cf. also Geller, *Renal and Rectal Disease Texts*, 177.

[93] *STT* I 97 iii: 15–18: *šumma amēlu šuburra-šú ḫa-niq-ma šuburra-šú ur-še um-ṣa-a-ti mali ana bulluṭī-šú* / *nīnâ burāša kanakta šammi balāṭi* / *mal-ma-liš ištēniš ina lipê u ḫīl baluḫḫi tuballal ubāna teppuš* / *ana šuburrī-šú tašakkan-ma iballuṭ*.

[94] Cf. Geller, *Renal and Rectal Disease Texts*, 130–131 l. 21.

[95] See his *Glass and Glassmaking in Ancient Mesopotamia* (Corning, NY: J.J. Agustin, 1970), 4.

proceedings are united, in others they are separated which is, in all likelihood, due to the fact that several strands of traditions were incorporated into the texts.

Further investigations will not only have to dwell upon nature and technical potential of the raw products available or on the individual preferences and social demands but also take into account the development and internal history of medical texts and their compilation into handbooks.

L'ANCIENNETÉ DE LA MÉDECINE HIPPOCRATIQUE : UN ESSAI DE BILAN

Paul Demont*

S'il est à l'heure actuelle difficile d'évaluer l'influence éventuelle de la médecine babylonienne sur la médecine grecque hippocratique, le développement considérable des études cunéiformes permet de prendre du recul par rapport à la tradition des études grecques, qui a construit dès l'antiquité l'image, à beaucoup d'égards inexacte, d'un Hippocrate à l'origine de la médecine occidentale. Dans la perspective d'une indispensable information mutuelle entre les deux spécialités, mon titre annonce un essai de bilan,—ajoutons : un essai de bilan partiel—, portant uniquement sur la médecine dite « hippocratique », c'est-à-dire réunie dans ce qu'il est convenu d'appeler la *Collection hippocratique* en partie dès l'antiquité, et en partie à l'époque médiévale. Cet essai de bilan tente, à partir de l'état des débats entre hellénistes, d'évaluer les critères leur permettant de faire l'histoire de cette médecine hippocratique, sur deux points : la nature de la polémique du traité de *La Maladie sacrée*, et les discussions autour des écoles médicales.

Les premiers à avoir appelé « sacrée » la Maladie sacrée : histoire interne et histoire externe de la médecine

> A mon avis, ceux qui les premiers ont attribué un caractère sacré à cette maladie étaient des gens comparables à ce que sont aujourd'hui encore mages, purificateurs, prêtres mendiants et charlatans, tous gens qui affectent d'être fort pieux et de détenir un savoir supérieur. (I, 4, VI 354 Li, 3–4 Jouanna, trad. J. Jouanna)

La polémique vigoureuse contre l'appellation de « maladie sacrée » qui donne son titre au traité (d'une façon exceptionnelle : c'est le seul traité

* Université de Paris-Sorbonne (Paris-IV).

hippocratique qui soit consacré à une seule maladie) a donné lieu récemment à des appréciations divergentes à l'intérieur même du monde des hellénistes.[1]

Le nom de « maladie sacrée » est employé dans un autre traité de la *Collection hippocratique* sans commentaire particulier[2]; dans deux autres, on trouve à la fois « maladie sacrée » et « maladie dite sacrée »[3]; enfin il existe deux attestations isolées de l'appellation « maladie dite sacrée ».[4] Platon associe lui aussi une formule modalisée et une formule sans modalisation, dans un texte des *Lois* relatif à la vente d'esclaves susceptibles d'être épileptiques.[5] Il justifie tant bien que mal l'appellation de « maladie sacrée » dans le *Timée*.[6] De nombreux textes juridiques emploient la formule sans modalisation.[7] Les deux expressions, l'expression qu'on définit comme traditionnelle, « maladie sacrée », et l'expression modalisée, « maladie dite sacrée », sont donc dans l'usage de la prose hippocratique, et peut-être de la prose en général, faute d'un terme technique remplaçant

---

[1] Les nouveaux textes babyloniens sur l'épilepsie—cf. J.V. Kinnier Wilson and E.H. Reynolds, « Texts and documents: Translation and analysis of a cuneiform text forming part of a babylonian treatise on epilepsy », *Medical History* 34 (1990): 185–198 et Marten Stol, *Epilepsy in Babylonia* Cuneiform Monographs 2 (Groningen: Styx Publication, 1993)—ne sont pas pris en considération dans Michael Wöhlers, *Heilige Krankheit, Epilepsie in antiker Medizin, Astrologie und Religion*, (Marburg: N.G. Elwert, 1999), ni dans Hippocrate, t. II, 3ème partie, *La Maladie sacrée*, texte établi et traduit par Jacques Jouanna (Paris: Les Belles Lettres (CUF), 2003). Sur leur mise en relation éventuelle, cf. Markham J. Geller, « West meets East: Early Greek and Babylonian Medicine », *Archiv für Orientforschung* 48/49, (2001–2002): 50–75 et JoAnn Scurlock, « From Esagil-kīn-apli to Hippocrates », *Le Journal des Médecines Cunéiformes* 3 (2004): 11–14.

[2] *Maladies des femmes* 151 (τἄλλα ὅcα οἱ ὑπὸ ἱερῆc νούcου ἐπίληπτοι πάcχουcι, 'tous les autres maux dont souffrent ceux qui sont saisis [*epileptoi*] par une maladie sacrée', Li VIII, 326).

[3] Cf. *Vents* 14.1 (VI, 110 Li 121 Jouanna : τὴν ἱρὴν καλεομένην νοῦcον) et 14.4 (112 Li 122 Jouanna : τὴν ἱρὴν νοῦcον), *Prorrhétique II* 5 (IX, 20 Li VIII, 234 Potter : ὑπὸ τῆc ἱερῆc νόcου καλεομένηc) et 9 (28 Li 242 ὑπὸ τῆc ἱερῆc νόcου).

[4] *Airs, Eaux, Lieux* 4 (II, 20 Li 194 Jouanna : τά τε ἱερὰ νοcεύματα καλεύμενα, cf. aussi 3.3, 191 Jouanna), *Maladies des jeunes filles* 1 (VIII, 466 Li 248 Flemming-Hanson : περὶ τῆc ἱερῆc νούcου καλεομένηc).

[5] Platon, *Lois*. XI, 916a6 : τῇ καλουμένῃ ἱερᾷ νόcῳ ἢ καὶ ἑτέρῳ τινὶ ἀδήλῳ τοῖc πολλοῖc. νοcήματι μακρῷ καὶ δυcιάτῳ κατὰ τὸ cῶμα ἢ κατὰ τὴν διάνοιαν et b5 : τῆc ἱερᾶc.

[6] Platon, *Timée*, 85b : la maladie, dit-il, touche ce qu'il y a de plus sacré en l'homme, la tête et le cerveau.

[7] Cf. l'excursus de Wöhlers, 122–126, sur cette expression : il donne n. 187 les références de nombreux textes papyrologiques concernant des ventes d'esclaves, où se trouve la formule πλὴν ἐπαφῆc καὶ ἱερᾶc νόcου (ou la formule inverse). Voir aussi l'édition de Jacques Jouanna [cf. n. 1], XXIII–XXIV.

les désignations traditionnelles. L'expression modalisée témoigne-t-elle, de la part de certains, comme le dit Jacques Jouanna à propos des médecins, d'un souci de «prendre leurs distances» par rapport à cette dénomination traditionnelle, qu'ils utilisent cependant aussi[8] ? C'est possible. On peut également penser, si on comprend «la maladie connue comme maladie sacrée», qu'elle indique seulement un autre nom de la «grande maladie», comme on l'appelle aussi.[9]

Hérodote, dès le milieu du cinquième siècle, emploie, à propos de la folie épileptique du roi Cambyse—l'épilepsie entre en effet le plus souvent en grec dans le tableau général de la folie—, une expression assez similaire, «la maladie que certains appellent sacrée» (τὴν ἱρὴν ὀνομάζουσί τινες, III, 33), sans préciser l'identité de ceux qui emploient ce nom. Peut-on voir chez lui un souci polémique comparable à celui du traité hippocratique de la *Maladie sacrée* et, avec Rosalind Thomas,[10] intégrer ainsi le traité hippocratique ou ses devanciers dans le « contexte » d'Hérodote ? Il n'est pas sûr, à mon sens, si l'on considère les emplois cités de cette formulation dans la *Collection hippocratique* et ailleurs, qu'on ait ici «a clear allusion» à la thèse précise défendue dans *la Maladie sacrée*; en revanche, dans le passage où il mentionne cette appellation, et si l'on se place d'un point de vue assez général, Hérodote, de fait, «is thinking along much the same lines» que les textes hippocratiques, «especially in the recognition of heredity, and the relation of physical ill-health and mental well-being».

Ce n'est pas le seul cas où Hérodote[11] atteste l'ancienneté de tel ou tel aspect de la médecine que nous connaissons comme hippocratique, et permet ainsi d'en montrer la diffusion au cinquième siècle, voire dès le

[8] Cf. *ibid.*, XXV. Le cas d'*Airs, Eaux, Lieux* c. III, 3 «les accidents que l'on dit provoquer la 'maladie de l'enfant' et être la maladie sacrée» (Hippocrate, t. II, 2ème partie, *Airs, Eaux, Lieux*, texte établi et traduit par Jacques Jouanna (Paris: Les Belles Lettres (CUF), 1996), 191), où l'auteur donne deux noms successifs qui sont attribués à cette maladie, «maladie de l'enfant» et «maladie sacrée», est néanmoins incertain, car le texte ne donne guère d'indication suggérant que « dans l'esprit de l'auteur, cette dénomination soit correcte dans le cas de τὸ παιδίον et incorrecte dans le cas de ἱερὴν νοῦσον» (Jouanna, *ad loc.* 260).

[9] Références dans Jouanna, *La Maladie* ..., XXV n. 37. Wöhlers, 126 observe la coexistence, à l'époque hellénistique, de deux interprétations de l'expression, l'une avec un sens religieux (critiqué notamment par Callimaque), l'autre avec un sens seulement technique : cette coexistence peut être plus ancienne.

[10] Rosalind Thomas, *Herodotus in Context. Ethnography, Science and Persuasion* (Cambridge: Cambridge U.P., 2000), 34–35.

[11] Il faudrait aussi mentionner les rapports entre la médecine hippocratique et le théâtre. Voir la synthèse récente d'Alessia Guardasole, *Tragedia e Medicina nell'Atene del V secolo A.C.* (Napoli: D'Auria Editore, 2000).

début du cinquième siècle. Wilhem Nestle l'a fait observer dès 1908 à propos de la doctrine du changement des saisons (μεταβολή) comme cause des maladies.[12] Mirko D. Grmek a comparé la description hérodotéenne de la guérison « en douceur » de la cheville de Darius par le médecin Démocédès de Crotone au traitement recommandé au c. 10 de *Fractures.*[13] J'ai attiré l'attention sur la juxtaposition, chez Hérodote, de descriptions traditionnelles des maladies pestilentielles et d'un *loimos* associé à une « dysenterie » avec une causalité évoquant *Ancienne médecine.*[14] Rosalind Thomas a proposé récemment une synthèse très bien informée dans le chapitre « Medecine and the ethnography of health » de son livre déjà cité. Notons ici seulement un point sur lequel je reviendrai : Hérodote connaît φλέγμα non pas avec le sens archaïque d'« incendie » ou « inflammation » qu'avait naturellement ce dérivé du verbe φλέγω « enflammer », mais avec le sens médical de « phlegme » ou « pituite », humeur descendant de la tête et causant des maladies, et il décrit les cautérisations que subissent, dès l'enfance, avec succès selon lui, les Libyens pour bloquer ces descentes de phlegme et être ainsi, peut-être pour cette raison (Hérodote est prudent), de tous les hommes, ceux qui jouissent de la meilleure santé, ce dont une autre cause, indiquée dans un autre livre, est aussi l'absence de changements brutaux dans les saisons (IV, 187[15] et II, 77). Or, inversement, le phlegme venant du cerveau est, dès la gestation et la petite enfance, la principale cause de la « maladie sacrée » selon l'auteur du traité hippocratique *Maladie sacrée*, et les changements

[12] Wilhem Nestle, « Herodots Verhältnis zur Philosophie und Sophistik », Programm des ev.-theol. Seminars in Schöntal, 1908 (Stuttgart: Druck der Stuttgarter Vereinsbuchdruckerei, 1908); « Gab es eine ionische Sophistik? », *Philologus* 70 (1911): 242–266, « Hippocratica, » *Hermes* 73, (1938): 23–28. Cf. aussi Jochen Althoff, « Herodot und die griechische Medizin, » *Antike Naturwissenschaft und ihre Rezeption*, herausgegeben von Klaus Döring und Georg Wöhrle, (Bamberg: Collibri Verlag, 1993), 1–16.

[13] « L'ancienneté de la chirurgie hippocratique », *Formes de pensée dans la Collection hippocratique : Actes du IVe colloque hippocratique international (Lausanne, 21–26 sept. 1981)*, éds. François Lasserre et Philippe Mudry (Genève: Droz, 1983), 285–296.

[14] Paul Demont, « Hérodote et les pestilences », *Revue de Philologie* 62 (1988): 7–13.

[15] « Les Libyens nomades en effet, sinon tous, ce que je ne puis dire avec certitude, du moins beaucoup d'entre eux, font ceci quand leurs enfants ont quatre ans, ils leur brûlent avec de la laine non dégraissée les veines du sommet de la tête, et quelques-uns celles des tempes, afin d'éviter pour toujours que la pituite s'écoule de leur tête et compromette leur santé; et c'est grâce à cela, prétendent-ils, qu'ils ont une excellente santé. En vérité, les Libyens sont, de tous les hommes que nous connaissons, les plus sains ; si c'est grâce à cette opération, je ne peux le dire avec certitude; mais le fait est qu'ils ont une santé excellente » (Hérodote, IV, 187, trad. Ph.-E. Legrand).

brusques du temps y sont une cause déclenchante importante. Hérodote n'évoque certes pas la « maladie sacrée » à propos de la Libye, mais on ne peut qu'être frappé de ce double parallélisme.[16]

Revenons à ce traité et à la construction du passé de la médecine par l'auteur lui-même. D'une façon exceptionnelle dans nos sources, l'appellation « maladie dite sacrée » lui permet de poser la question de l'origine de ce nom de « maladie sacrée », dans la phrase que j'ai citée pour commencer. Quand l'auteur attribue à des individus précis et situe dans le passé (« ceux qui les premiers ont ... ») l'invention de ce nom, se livrant ainsi à « una storia della sacralizzazione della malattia », s'il se conforme à l'habitude fréquente dans la pensée grecque du cinquième siècle qui consiste à rechercher un « premier inventeur » à toutes choses, qu'il s'agisse de techniques ou de croyances, la phrase a une intention rhétorique inhabituelle, car, au lieu de célébrer ces premiers inventeurs, elle les vitupère et les « assimile à une série de contemporains peu recommandables ».[17] Le procédé permet, d'une part, de ne pas attaquer de front l'opinion populaire ou traditionnelle en général, mais seulement un groupe restreint d'individus du passé, et, d'autre part, comme le tableau de ce groupe d'individus du passé est construit à l'aide d'une comparaison avec des contemporains, l'auteur peut par ce biais attaquer en même temps directement un certain nombre de ses contemporains.

Commençons par la recherche des premiers inventeurs. La méthode consistant, dans un traité médical, à présenter une histoire de la médecine est attestée en particulier dans l'*Ancienne médecine*. Les différences avec *Maladie sacrée* sont importantes. Dans *Ancienne médecine*, l'auteur remonte dans le temps, à partir de la médecine actuelle qui soigne les malades jusqu'à l'époque de son invention, et « en remontant encore plus haut » (III, 3),[18] à partir de l'invention de cette médecine des malades

---

[16] *Maladie sacrée* mentionne aussi cette bonne santé des Libyens : critiquant l'interdiction de manger de la viande de chèvre que certains proposent comme traitement à la maladie sacrée, l'auteur note que si cette interdiction était nécessaire à la santé, « aucun Libyen ne serait en bonne santé » (*Maladie sacrée* I, 6, VI, 356 Li 5 Jouanna :᾽Εγὼ δὲ δοκέω Λιβύων ἂν τῶν τὴν μεσόγειον οἰκεόντων οὐδέν᾽ ἂν ὑγιαίνειν, avec la note 5 p. 48 de Jouanna sur l'histoire de l'établissement du texte, qui a longtemps été compris, à tort, en un sens opposé).

[17] Cf. Amneris Roselli in Ippocrate, *La malattia sacra*, a c. di A.R., con testo a fronte (Venezia: Marsilio, 1996), n. 6 p. 90 (citant H.-W. Nörenberg, *Das Göttliche und die Natur in der Schrift Über die heilige Krankheit*, (Bonn: Habelt—Germany, 1968), 28) et Jacques Jouanna, n. 8 p. 38.

[18] ἔτι δὲ ἄνωθεν... Je cite la traduction de Jacques Jouanna dans : Hippocrate, t. II, 1ère partie, *L'ancienne médecine*, texte établi et traduit par Jacques Jouanna, Paris, Les

jusqu'à l'invention préalable de l'art de la santé. Il tient à faire de cette invention, qui est en fait celle de l'art de faire le pain,[19] plutôt que l'art de la cuisine, une sorte de première médecine, comme il le dit explicitement : « A cette découverte et à cette enquête, quel nom plus juste ou plus adéquat pourrait-on donner que celui de médecine, puisqu'il s'agit d'une découverte faite pour la santé, le salut et la nourriture de l'homme ? ».[20] La description historique a pour fonction ici d'étendre dans le passé le royaume de la médecine, et de critiquer par la même occasion ceux qui prétendent inventer une nouvelle médecine fondée sur des « postulats » au lieu de l'observation et de l'analyse des affections des malades. En revanche, dans *Maladie sacrée*, qu'il s'agisse des premiers inventeurs ou des contemporains, l'auteur du traité hippocratique évite, dans tout le prologue, d'appeler « médecins » et de parler de « médecine » à propos de l'appellation « maladie sacrée ». Son traité propose donc une rupture et non une continuité. Ces gens qui dans le passé ont inventé le nom de « maladie sacrée » n'apparaissent pas du tout, de son point de vue, comme des collègues ayant autrefois partagé la même *technè* que la sienne.

De même, les contemporains auxquels ils sont comparés n'ont, pour lui, rien à voir avec la médecine, puisqu'ils sont « mages, purificateurs, prêtres mendiants et charlatans », mots qu'on ne trouve pas ailleurs dans la *Collection hippocratique*.[21] Le dernier mot, ἀλαζόνες, « charlatans », c'est-à-dire « faux savants », prépare directement le verbe de la relative qui suit, προσποιέονται « qui affectent de ... », et oriente le sens de l'ensemble de la liste : l'auteur montrera, contrairement à ses adversaires, le vrai sens de la piété religieuse et la véritable nature de la maladie dite sacrée. Les trois autres termes renvoient plus nettement aux rites religieux, avec un terme qui est employé de façon positive dans le théâtre classique,[22] καθάρται, « purificateurs », et deux termes dépréciatifs, associés comme tels chez Sophocle lorsque le roi Œdipe insulte le devin Tirésias, μάγοι,

Belles Lettres (CUF), 1990; sur « l'archéologie » de la médecine, voir son analyse pp. 34–49. Voir aussi son étude : « La naissance de l'histoire de la médecine en Grèce à l'époque classique », *Histoire des Sciences Médicales*, (*Centenaire de la Société Française d'Histoire de la Médecine, 1902–2002, Paris, 29 et 30 novembre 2002*), t. 37, n°3 (2003), 319–329.

[19] « A partir des grains de blé, après les avoir mouillés, mondés, moulus, tamisés, pétris et cuits, ils confectionnèrent le pain, et à partir des grains d'orge, la galette » (I, 576 Li 121 Jouanna).

[20] II, 6 (I, 578 Li 123 Jouanna).

[21] Voir en dernier lieu Jacques Jouanna, p. XXVIII–XIX (comparaison avec *Œdipe-Roi*, v. 387–388) et 38–40 (avec bibliographie) et Marcello Carastro, *La cité des mages. Penser la magie en Grèce ancienne* (Grenoble: Ed. J. Millon, 2006), 43–53.

[22] Sophocle, *Electre* 70, Aristophane, *Guêpes* 1043.

« mages » sur lequel je reviendrai, et ἀγύρται, qui signifie « mendiants » (notamment sous le patronage d'une divinité) et dont le second est associé aussi de façon très péjorative à μάντεις « devins » par Platon dans la *République*.[23] Cette polémique « passionnée », dont « l'âpreté » (J. Jouanna) frappe tout lecteur, a été interprétée de diverses façons par les hellénistes. Je mentionnerai rapidement trois orientations récentes.

On a eu beau jeu, malgré cette polémique spectaculaire, de rapprocher la médecine hippocratique de la médecine « magico-religieuse », de contester, donc, la qualification de « médecine rationnelle » qui lui est appliquée de nos jours, et de suggérer enfin que, dans la polémique de *Maladie sacrée*, la supériorité intellectuelle de l'auteur du traité sur ses adversaires est douteuse. Robert Parker, par exemple, notamment à partir des travaux d'O. Temkin, de F. Kudlien et de G. Lloyd, mais aussi de Dietlinde Goltz, qu'il est un des rares hellénistes à utiliser,[24] décrit à ce propos, et de façon plus générale, les ressemblances de famille entre la médecine hippocratique et la médecine magico-religieuse à propos de l'usage de la *katharsis*, des *pharmaka*, des bains et des fumigations, dans le chapitre « Disease, Bewitchment and Purifiers » de son *Miasma*,[25] tout en notant que « the original family likeness is simply not perceived » par les médecins hippocratiques. Cette notation est insuffisante : on devrait dire plutôt qu'elle est explicitement déniée.

Un peu avant que paraisse l'édition de Jacques Jouanna, Julie Laskaris est allée plus loin.[26] Elle a d'abord le mérite de rappeler les témoignages les plus anciens, indépendants de la littérature, et donc le plus souvent négligés par les hellénistes, sur la médecine grecque : ce sont notamment l'attestation de l'attribution d'un lot de terre, probablement pour services rendus, à un *i-ja-te*, c'est-à-dire d'un ἰατήρ, en mycénien, sur une tablette de Pylos (*PY Eq* 146, antérieure à 1200 avant J.-C.),[27] la découverte d'instruments médicaux de bonne qualité dans une tombe de

---

[23] Sophocle, *Œdipe-Roi*, v. 387–388, Platon, *République*, II, 364 b-c.

[24] Dietlinde Goltz, *Studien zur altorientalischen und griechischen Heilkunde: Therapie, Arzneibereitung, Rezeptstruktur*, (Wiesbaden: Franz Steiner Verlag, 1974).

[25] Robert Parker, *Miasma: Pollution and Purification in Early Greek Religion* (Oxford: Clarendon, 1983), 207–234.

[26] *The Art is Long. On the Sacred Disease and the Scientific Tradition* (Leiden: Brill, 2002) (pp. 62–72 sur la réception « moderne », avec notamment une distinction remarquable entre l'idée de Wilamowitz d'une conception scientifique de la religion chez le médecin et l'opinion d'Edelstein et d'elle-même selon laquelle l'unité de la causalité naturelle et de la causalité divine dans le traité est « fairly conventional »).

[27] M. Ventris et J. Chadwick, *Documents in Mycenaean Greek*, 1973^2, Cambridge, 547. Ce texte est absent du précieux recueil d'Evelyne Samama, *Les médecins dans le monde*

l'âge du bronze à Nauplies (1450–1400 avant J.-C.) et des cas de trépanation réussie dès l'âge du bronze ; elle mentionne aussi, à partir d'études d'ethnobotanistes, le rôle joué, dans la médecine des herbes, par la notion de saveur (en particulier l'amertume)—une notion attestée largement dans la littérature grecque, de l'*Iliade*, où elle conserve une valeur magico-religieuse (11, 846), à Théophraste,[28] et surtout, je voudrais y insister, une notion qui est inséparable de la notion hippocratique « d'humeur ».[29] En ce qui concerne proprement *Maladie sacrée*, l'auteur du traité, souligne-t-elle, ne cherche nullement « to distinguish science from magic on a theoretical basis », et donc ne fait jamais aucun développement sur la causalité naturelle : il cherche seulement à montrer que ses adversaires ne respectent pas la piété, entendue dans un sens tout à fait conventionnel (« we should bear in mind that no conventionally pious Greek would have considered the forces of nature to be anything but divine »[30]). L'objectif principalement rhétorique qu'a le traité selon elle explique aussi, par exemple, qu'au cours du développement final sur le cerveau, une place soit laissée à la bile comme cause de la folie, alors que le traité repose sur une explication de la maladie sacrée par le phlegme : il fallait tenir compte de l'association traditionnelle entre épilepsie et folie, et entre folie et bile. Même la conception héréditaire de la maladie ne relève pas exclusivement de la causalité naturelle : « as far as his audience is concerned, the author's genetic argument is not proof at all that the disease is not god-sent ».[31] Dans cette interprétation, donc, la polémique est inscrite à l'intérieur d'une société où les médecins de diverses obédiences sont en compétition farouche, dans le cadre général de la piété traditionnelle, par rapport auquel l'auteur a bien du mal à soutenir une originalité qui ne réside guère dans la rationalité des analyses proposées.

---

grec. Sources épigraphiques sur la naissance d'un corps médical (Genève: Droz, 2003), limité au grec alphabétique, ce qui donne une idée inexacte de la « naissance » d'un corps médical.

[28] Voir aussi Platon, *République*, IV, 426a–b.

[29] Sur les rapports entre « humeur » et « saveur », je me permets de renvoyer à mon étude « About philosophy and humoural medicine, » *Hippocrates in Context, Papers read at the XIth International Hippocrates Colloquium, University of Newcastle upon Tyne (27–31 August 2002)*, éd. Ph. J. Van der Eijk (Leiden: Brill, 2005), 271–286. Dans une perspective différente, Jacques Jouanna et moi-même avons essayé de montrer l'ancienneté de la notion hippocratique d'*ichôr* à partir des célèbres emplois du mot dans l'*Iliade* à propos du sang des dieux (« Le sens d'ἰχώρ chez Homère et Eschyle en relation avec les emplois du mot dans la Collection hippocratique », *Revue des Etudes Anciennes* 83 (1981): 197–209).

[30] P. 122.

[31] P. 148.

Dans sa récente édition, Jacques Jouanna offre, lui, la version la plus documentée et la plus précise de l'interprétation traditionnelle, selon laquelle l'auteur du traité défend une médecine « rationnelle » contre une médecine « magico-religieuse ». Il caractérise la « médecine rationnelle » par la « grande importance » manifestement accordée dans le traité « à la notion de cause » : origine innée, processus internes semblables pour tous, causes externes, en particulier environnementales.[32] En second lieu, cette médecine rationnelle lui apparaît, comme auparavant à Wilamowitz, proposer une conception « épurée » de la divinité, qui laisse cependant sa place à la médecine des grands sanctuaires, explicitement mentionnée.[33] En ce qui concerne la médecine « magico-religieuse », ses analyses et ses procédés, tels qu'ils sont décrits dans le traité, relèvent à la fois de la « possession » par une divinité reconnue dans la religion traditionnelle[34] et de règlements diététiques attestés notamment dans les conseils des Pythagoriciens. Mais Jacques Jouanna montre clairement aussi que cette médecine « a pu rivaliser avec la médecine rationnelle », premièrement en faisant « des distinctions fines entre les symptômes pour y faire correspondre des variétés de maladies », selon un principe qu'on retrouve dans les traités nosologiques de la *Collection hippocratique*, et qui remonte, selon Jacques Jouanna, à la « médecine cnidienne » (la différence, « fondamentale » à ses yeux, étant que la médecine de ces traités rattache ces maladies à la nature et non à des puissances divines[35]), et en second lieu, en traitant le malade avec des interdits

---

[32] P. XXXIX–XLVIII.

[33] P. XXXVII. Dans cette médecine des sanctuaires, la divinité « est ce qui purifie, ce qui sanctifie, notre nettoyant » (I, 13, VI, 364 Li 9 Jouanna avec la n. 6 de J. Jouanna). Comme le note Philip J. van der Eijk (« The Theology of the Hippocratic Treatise *On the Sacred Disease* », *Apeiron* 23 (1990): 87–119, 111), « cleansing is performed by the *divine*, not (as the magicians believe) by human beings ». Cette croyance, avérée, en des dieux purificateurs dans les sanctuaires où on les honore par des prières et des sacrifices, d'un côté, et l'identification entre le caractère divin et le caractère naturel de la maladie, de l'autre, sont compatibles si l'on se souvient que « the borderlines between secular medicine and temple-medicine were vague and the relationship between these was seldom hostile or antagonistic » (117).

[34] Wesley D. Smith, « So-called Possession in Pre-Christian Greece » (*Transactions and Proceedings of the American Philological Association* 96 (1965): 403–426) attire avec raison l'attention sur la différence entre la « possession » par les « démons » dans la démonologie chrétienne et l'attaque de l'homme par certaines divinités dans la religion grecque (voir aussi Wöhlers [cf. n. 1], pp. 121–122 sur le sens de τὸ δαιμόνιον dans *Maladie sacrée* I, 27), mais il paraît néanmoins difficile de ne pas employer le vocabulaire de la « possession » dans les deux cas (notamment pour traduire ἔνθεος, cf. par ex. Euripide, *Hippolyte*, 141–148, qui a été souvent rapproché, avec raison, de *Maladie sacrée*, cf. Jouanna, p. XXXII).

[35] P. XXXIII.

alimentaires dont l'auteur de *Maladie sacrée* lui-même reconnaît que certains sont fondés du point de vue du régime, et non de la religion (I, 4).[36] L'interprétation de Jacques Jouanna présente donc, dans une perspective évolutionniste, le traité comme « le premier témoignage conservé sur la naissance de la médecine rationnelle », tout en discernant dans la médecine dite « magico-religieuse » vitupérée, dans sa différence par rapport à la médecine miraculeuse des sanctuaires, certains aspects proches de la nosologie attestée dans les traités les plus anciens de la *Collection hippocratique*.

Signalons enfin une troisième attitude à l'égard de ce traité, plus récente encore, un peu marginale par rapport à notre sujet, mais qui pose une question de fond. Marcello Carastro vient de consacrer un livre à la création en grec, à l'époque classique, de la notion de *mageia*. Bien que cette notion soit formée à partir du mot iranien *magos*, dont les Grecs connaissaient le sens, comme en témoigne Hérodote, elle est uniquement, estime-t-il, un « produit culturel grec »,[37] et doit être considérée comme tel pour éviter les controverses sur la magie et la religion, les risques d'un recours à une conception ontologique de la magie tout autant que ceux d'une approche que les anthropologues appellent « étique », c'est-à-dire fondée surtout sur les catégories de l'observateur. La mention des mages dans le traité *Maladie sacrée* est lue dans cette perspective, au moyen des études antérieures, notamment celle de Giuliana Lanata[38] : cette mention ne peut pas, selon lui, être une allusion aux *magoi* iraniens, mais seulement un moyen, par la création d'une notion grecque du « mage », de critiquer les « guérisseurs traditionnels grecs ». Cette position anthropologique aboutit à exclure pour ainsi dire *a priori* la possibilité d'un emprunt, ce qui paraît excessif, quel que soit l'intérêt des remarques sur l'élaboration proprement grecque de la « magie » et ses conséquences dans les mentalités occidentales.

La situation à l'intérieur même du monde des hellénistes, avant même qu'ils prennent conscience de la possibilité d'une influence babylonienne, ou en tout cas de la nécessité d'une comparaison, est donc complexe. Ajoutons un dernier mot sur *Maladie sacrée*. La thérapeutique en est quasiment absente, si l'on excepte quelques rapides considérations générales sur le régime à donner, dans le dernier chapitre. Ces brèves considéra-

[36] P. XXXI.
[37] Carastro, *La cité des mages* ..., 9.
[38] Giulana Lanata, *Medicina magica e religione popolare in Grecia fino all' età di Ippocrate*, (Roma: Ateneo, 1967).

tions font curieusement écho aux aspects diététiques de la médecine des thérapeutes religieux, aspects auxquels l'auteur concédait une certaine validité, mais d'un point de vue diététique et non pas religieux, au début de l'œuvre: si l'auteur est si rapide, c'est peut-être pour ne pas avoir à reconnaître cette part commune. De fait, la diététique est généralement présentée plutôt comme une *innovation* décisive des médecins modernes dans *Ancienne Médecine* et ailleurs,[39] et Platon confirme, en la condamnant, cette façon de faire l'histoire de la médecine grecque ancienne dans sa fameuse opposition du livre III (405c sqq.) de la *République* entre la médecine vertueuse, qui purge, cautérise ou incise, et la condamnable médecine moderne, qui prolonge inutilement et vicieusement la vie à coup de régimes compliqués.

Rédactions parallèles, couches de rédaction et écoles médicales

Du point de vue platonicien, *Maladie sacrée* représenterait donc une médecine moderne. Elle est pourtant ancienne par rapport à d'autres traités de la *Collection hippocratique*. J'en viens maintenant à la deuxième question que je voudrais présenter brièvement, celle de la datation relative, à l'époque moderne, des traités hippocratiques les uns par rapport aux autres.

Les critères très généraux qui ont été construits au dix-neuvième siècle apparaissent ainsi, si on reprend les dénominations de Louis Bourgey, un acteur décisif, avec Jacques Jouanna, de la renaissance des études hippocratiques[40]: il distingue «les médecins théoriciens», «les médecins à tendance empirique» et «les médecins d'esprit positif». Se distinguant de la médecine théorique, la *Collection hippocratique* serait essentiellement l'oeuvre des deux dernières catégories, que l'on devrait assimiler respectivement aux deux écoles rivales des Asclépiades de Cnide, l'école «empirique» plus ancienne, et des Asclépiades de Cos, l'école plus récente, «d'esprit positif».

---

[39] Notamment *Régime des Maladies aiguës*, 3 («Les anciens n'ont rien écrit de notable non plus à propos du régime, et ce fut une grave omission», II, 226 Li 37 Joly, référence de l'ouvrage note 44).

[40] Louis Bourgey, *Observation et expérience chez les médecins de la Collection hippocratique*, (Paris: Vrin, 1953). Ces dénominations sont empruntées à Emile Littré et à ses successeurs, en particulier allemands. Nous laissons ici de côté les questions relatives aux «médecins théoriciens».

Les années 1970 ont été décisives dans l'évolution de cette question, et un bref rappel de cette histoire récente est peut-être utile. D'un côté, Hermann Grensemann et Jacques Jouanna, travaillant en rapport mutuel, se sont consacrés à l'étude philologique extrêmement approfondie des témoignages sur l'école dite de Cnide, des rédactions parallèles et des couches de rédaction de l'ensemble appelé traditionnellement « cnidien », ce qui renforçait considérablement le soubassement concret de la notion d'école de Cnide.[41] Les travaux de Hermann Grensemann furent utilisés notamment par Dietlinde Goltz. De l'autre côté, dans les mêmes années, dans le monde anglo-saxon, Iain Lonie et Wesley Smith ont fait l'historiographie de la distinction entre école de Cnide et école de Cos et ont montré à quel point elle était liée au contexte de chaque époque, notamment, pour ne mentionner que deux moments et deux noms essentiels, à la lutte de Galien contre le méthodisme et au positivisme d'Emile Littré,[42] ce qui, inversement, limitait considérablement le bien-fondé et l'utilité de la distinction entre deux écoles rivales.[43] Les « Colloques hippocratiques » successifs qui se sont réunis depuis cette décennie montrent l'évolution des débats, parfois très vifs, entre les deux orientations.[44] Les deux ouvrages les plus importants sur le sujet sont peut-être l'édition du traité *Maladies II* procurée en 1983 par Jacques Jouanna, à laquelle il convient de se référer, où il reprend ses analyses antérieures en les nuançant parfois[45] et la synthèse de Volker Langholf, *Medical Theories in Hippocrates: Early Texts and the Epidemics*, qui reprend et élargit à son tour la critique de la notion d'école de Cnide,

[41] Jacques Jouanna, *Hippocrate: Pour une archéologie de l'école de Cnide*, (Paris: Les Belles Lettres, 1974); Hermann Grensemann, *Knidische Medizin: Teil I*, (Berlin/New York: De Gruyter, 1975); *Knidische Medizin: Teil II*, Hermes Einzelschriften Heft 51 (Stuttgart: Frantz Steiner, 1987).

[42] Cf. l'expression employée par Louis Bourgey: « les médecins d'esprit positif », pour définir l'école de Cos.

[43] Iain M. Lonie, « Hippocrates and the Historians. Cos versus Cnidus and the historians, » *History of Science* 16 (1978): 42–75 et 77–92, Wesley D. Smith, « Galen on Coans versus Cnidians, » *Bulletin of History of Medicine* 47 (1973): 569–585; *The Hippocratic Tradition* (Ithaca/London: Cornell UP, 1979).

[44] Voir en particulier *Corpus Hippocraticum : Actes du colloque hippocratique de Mons*, Mons, 1977, édités par Robert Joly, un des critiques les plus sévères (et les plus polémiques—ce qui a parfois trop limité l'attention portée à ses arguments) à l'égard des travaux de H. Grensemann et de J. Jouanna (voir notamment « L'école médicale de Cnide et son évolution », *L'Antiquité classique* 47 (1978): 528–537). Autre présentation critique, plus nuancée, dans Antoine Thivel, *Cnide et Cos ? Essai sur les doctrines médicales dans la Collection hippocratique* (Paris: Les Belles Lettres, 1981).

[45] Hippocrate, t. X, 2ème partie, *Maladies II*, texte établi et traduit par Jacques Jouanna (Paris: Les Belles Lettres CUF, 1983), 29–50. 29–50.

tout en acceptant les conclusions de H. Grensemann et de J. Jouanna sur la chronologie relative des traités hippocratiques.[46] Il est évidemment impossible de résumer en quelques minutes ces débats.

Rappelons du moins un texte essentiel, le début du traité hippocratique *Régime des maladies aiguës*, qui nous ramène encore une fois à la façon dont les médecins de l'époque classique construisaient l'histoire de la médecine. Cette fois, il ne s'agit pas pour cet auteur d'étendre la médecine à l'art de la santé en général, comme dans *Ancienne médecine*, ni de restreindre la médecine en excluant les guérisseurs traditionnels, comme dans *Maladie sacrée*, mais de se situer à l'intérieur même de la médecine. L'auteur, à la première personne, critique un ouvrage qu'il attribue à un groupe de médecins originaires de Cnide et qui contenait des descriptions de maladies avec un pronostic et une thérapeutique (1–2); il critique aussi « ceux qui par la suite ont remanié le traité », bien qu'ils aient fait, accorde-t-il, des progrès dans les prescriptions (3, 1).[47] L'un des auteurs de la *Collection hippocratique* déclare donc disposer d'ouvrages collectifs antérieurs, dans au moins deux versions différentes et successives, ouvrages par rapport auxquels il se faisait fort d'apporter du nouveau. Or les textes hippocratiques réunis dans la *Collection hippocratique* contiennent de très nombreux passages parallèles, parfois strictement identiques, parfois avec des modifications plus ou moins importantes, d'une oeuvre à l'autre, ou même à l'intérieur d'une même oeuvre (notamment dans le traité *Maladies II* où les mêmes maladies sont décrites deux fois, la première fois avec une étiologie humorale, la seconde fois sans étiologie, mais avec des indications thérapeutiques absentes de la première partie). Une grande partie du travail philologique a donc tout naturellement consisté à étudier ces rédactions parallèles dans la perspective historique qu'autorise manifestement ce texte, à l'intérieur notamment de deux grands groupes de rédactions parallèles, celui des traités nosologiques, et celui des *Epidémies*. On peut tenter d'expliquer d'une façon concrète, et complexe, ces désordres « anciens » dans les textes conservés : comme le rappelle, à la suite de Volker Langholf, Jacques Jouanna dans son édition d'*Epidémies V et VII* (où apparaissent aussi des rédactions

[46] Volker Langholf, *Medical Theories in Hippocrates: Early Texts and the Epidemics* (Berlin/New York: De Gruyter, 1990), 12–36 et 52 note 54.

[47] Cf. Hippocrate, t. VI, 2ème partie, *Du régime des maladies aiguës, Appendice, De l'aliment, De l'usage des liquides*, texte établi et traduit par Robert Joly (Paris: Les Belles Lettres CUF, 1972), 36–37. Voir aussi Hippocrate, *Du Régime*, texte établi et traduit par Robert Joly (Paris: Les Belles Lettres CUF, 1967), 1–2, avec l'analyse de Jacques Jouanna, « La naissance ... » (cité n°18).

parallèles), « on a supposé, de façon séduisante, l'existence d'archives à date ancienne où les textes médicaux, surtout quand ils étaient à usage interne, étaient copiés sur des pages de parchemin ou de papyrus (ou sur des tablettes de cire ou de bois), ce qui a pu favoriser les interversions ou les recompositions », qui ne sont pas toujours dues au hasard seulement et où le rôle « d'un épitomateur » est possible, « encore que ce terme puisse recouvrir des interventions faites à différentes étapes de la transmission ».[48]

Comment remettre de l'ordre ? Jacques Jouanna a entrepris cette tâche pour les traités *Maladies II* (qui comprend une double rédaction des mêmes maladies, les chapitres 1 à 11 étant repris à partir du chapitre 12 avec des rédactions parallèles), *Affections*, *Affections internes*, *Maladies I* et *Maladies III*, qui présentent entre eux et avec *Maladies II* d'autres rédactions parallèles, afin d'isoler des textes anciens et des textes récents, les plus anciens étant, selon ses conclusions, ceux de la deuxième partie du traité *Maladies II*. Hermann Grensemann est allé plus loin, en étudiant les traités gynécologiques, qui conservent les recettes médicales les plus étranges de la *Collection hippocratique* et qui sont encore actuellement relativement négligés[49] : c'est à l'intérieur même des rédactions parallèles qu'il a distingué trois couches de rédaction qu'il a nommées par ordre chronologique A, B et C, en alternant critères lexicaux (par exemple, selon le mot employé pour désigner les règles, καταμήνια ou ἐπιμήνια) et critères de plus ou moins grande proximité avec le schéma supposé le plus ancien de description des maladies dans l'ensemble des traités nosologiques.

Le point décisif est bien sûr la méthode adoptée pour déterminer les états anciens. Les critères utilisés peuvent être classés schématiquement en deux rubriques. D'un côté, il y a la reconstruction d'un modèle médical ancien qui serait un « écrit collectif des médecins de Cnide », selon l'expression de Jacques Jouanna,[50] à partir des témoignages galéniques sur les *Sentences cnidiennes*, sur les « médecins cnidiens » en général et d'une citation galénique du médecin Euryphon de Cnide qui est très semblable

---

[48] Hippocrate, t. IV, 3ème partie, *Epidémies V et VII*, texte établi et traduit par Jacques Jouanna (Paris: Les Belles Lettres CUF, 2000), XXXVI–XXXVII, citant notamment une communication de V. Langholf au colloque de Mons mentionné note 44.

[49] Voir Laskaris, *The Art* …, 6 et 16 sur les réticences des hellénistes à affronter ces textes avec renvoi aux travaux novateurs d'Ann Hanson et d'Heinrich von Staden. Voir cependant, tout récemment, Hippocrate, t. XII, 1ère partie, *Nature de la femme*, texte établi et traduit par Florence Bourbon (Paris: Les Belles Lettres CUF, 2008).

[50] Dans son édition de 1983, p. 48.

au chapitre 68 du traité *Maladies II* : cette reconstruction, que Jacques Jouanna juge toujours vraisemblable, Volker Langholf estime que, après les critiques qui en ont été faites, elle ne peut « neither be refuted nor proved correct », car elle est à son avis fondée sur des témoignages galéniques trop fragiles et incomplets.[51] De l'autre côté, il y a la comparaison entre les différentes rédactions et leur classement chronologique indépendamment de toute appartenance d'école, dont le même Volker Langholf reconnaît la validité.

Dans ce classement chronologique, on a parfois cherché des critères externes. Ainsi, Antoine Thivel, qui par ailleurs n'accepte pas la distinction entre Cos et Cnide, reprend, non sans hésitation, une remarque de Carl Fredrich selon laquelle les mesures utilisées dans la *Collection hippocratique* sont tantôt des mesures éginétiques, tantôt des mesures attiques, tantôt un système mixte.[52] Hermann Grensemann signale que Cnide a adhéré à l'empire athénien après la victoire grecque de la seconde guerre médique en 480–479 et donc dû adopter vers cette époque un système attique.[53] Cela donnerait une indication sur l'origine très ancienne, du tout début du cinquième siècle, de certains passages des traités gynécologiques « cnidiens ». Mais le système de mesure éginétique est en vigueur encore dans tout le quatrième siècle un peu partout en Grèce, comme on le voit, en matière monétaire, dans le corpus des inscriptions delphiques, et, en matière de poids, dans les inscriptions d'Olympie.[54] Les textes médicaux en question ayant été manifestement en usage aussi à cette date, et probablement dans le cadre d'une médecine itinérante dont les attaches avec Cnide sont incertaines, il n'y a rien de surprenant à ce double système, et probablement, à mon avis, rien d'utilisable pour une datation.

D'autres arguments ont été avancés. Revenons au traité *Maladie sacrée*. Deux critères tout à fait objectifs permettent de le situer à une période dite ancienne, c'est-à-dire au cinquième siècle: le critère du vocabulaire (le traité ne comporte pas l'adjectif *epileptikos*, « épileptique », qui est connu des *Aphorismes* et d'Aristote) et le critère humoral (si la bile intervient, comme on l'a vu, en quelque sorte par raccroc, le traité ne mentionne pas, dans les causes de l'épilepsie, la bile noire, à la différence, encore,

---

[51] Langholf, *Medical* ..., 22.
[52] Thivel, *Cnide et* ..., 94.
[53] Grensemann, *Knidische* ..., 50.
[54] Cf. e. g., pour Delphes, *CID* 10, et pour Olympie, *SEG* LI, 556, XLVII, 451, XLIX, 484.

des *Aphorismes*, d'*Epidémies VI* et du corpus aristotélicien).[55] Ces deux critères peuvent être réunis: le mot «mélancolie» (μελαγχολία) ou les mots apparentés font, pour nous, leur entrée dans la langue grecque chez le poète comique Aristophane, en 414 avant notre ère, avec un sens traditionnel proche de «folie», et l'on peut situer vers la même époque les traités hippocratiques où la notion de «maladie mélancolique» est constituée.[56] A côté de la question de la bile noire, la présence ou non de la doctrine des «crises» a été explorée à nouveau récemment de façon très fructueuse par Volker Langholf.[57]

Il n'en reste pas moins que le maniement de ces critères n'est pas toujours aisé. Après la bile, évoquons un peu plus longuement le phlegme. Un exemple concret des rédactions parallèles des traités nosologiques permettra de juger sur pièces, et de revenir aussi aux premiers textes évoqués aujourd'hui. Le mot φλέγμα qui a le sens d'«incendie» chez Homère, a encore parfois le sens d'«inflammation» chez Hippocrate selon Galien, tout en ayant aussi, bien sûr, le plus souvent, le sens humoral de «phlegme», humeur froide venant du cerveau. Pour dater l'une par rapport à l'autre les deux parties de *Maladies II*, Jacques Jouanna utilise les emplois de φλέγμα de deux façons. D'une part, en observant dans la seconde partie la survivance du sens ancien d'«inflammation», d'autre part, en opposant à la seconde partie, sans étiologie humorale, la première partie, avec étiologie humorale (notamment par le phlegme). Examinons ces deux aspects successivement.

«Dans la seconde partie, observe-t-il, φλέγμα a, dans la majorité des cas, le sens d'"inflammation' ou de 'gonflement inflammatoire'», alors que dans la première partie, le mot «désigne incontestablement une humeur froide».[58] Cette observation a été critiquée pour deux raisons principales, qui ne sont pas sur le même plan. Puisque c'est seulement «dans la majorité des cas» que le sens d'inflammation est reconnu, il est surprenant

---

55 Cf. Jacques Jouanna, p. XXV n. 36 et L n. 77. La «bile noire» comme entité autonome apparaît pour la première fois dans le traité *De la nature de l'homme* du médecin Polybe, qui était probablement le gendre d'Hippocrate. Cf. HIPPOCRATIS *De natura hominis*, par Jacques Jouanna (Corpus Medicorum Graecorum I, 1, 3), Berlin, 2002[2] (1975), addenda pp. 335–336.

56 Cf. Langholf, *Medical* . . ., 46–50 et 267–269, renvoyant à Walter Müri, «Melancholie und schwarze Galle,» Museum Helveticum 10 (1953), 21–38, in *Antike Medizin*, ed. von Hellmut Flashar, Wege der Forschung 121 (Darmstadt: Wissenschaftliche Buchgesellschaft, 1971), 165–191. et à Hellmut Flashar, *Melancholie und Melancholiker in den medizinischen Theorien der Antike* (Berlin: W. De Gruyter, 1966).

57 Langholf, *Medical* . . ., chap. III.

58 Jouanna, *Hippocrate. Pour une* . . ., 96.

que le mot puisse avoir dans le même traité deux sens si différents. Mais les deux sens sont-ils absolument incompatibles ? L'appellation φλέγμα λευκόν qui désigne la maladie décrite au c. 71, et que Jacques Jouanna traduit dans son édition par « Leucophlegmasie » peut se référer à la fois à un gonflement inflammatoire et à une collection de l'humeur phlegme.[59] Emile Littré dans son *Dictionnaire de la langue française* (éd. de 1883) s.v. « anasarque » cite Ambroise Paré : « Quand toute l'habitude du corps est pleine de phlegme blanc, on appelle l'hydropisie anasarca ou leucophlegmatia ». Pour le médecin du seizième siècle, comme pour Littré, il y a, semble-t-il, compatibilité entre gonflement inflammatoire et gonflement de phlegme blanc. Selon l'attitude que l'on adopte à l'égard de ce critère sémantique, on sera donc plus ou moins convaincu par la démonstration de Jacques Jouanna.

Le second critère tient à l'absence de l'étiologie humorale dans la seconde partie de *Maladies II*, qui remonterait donc à une époque antérieure à la systématisation de l'opposition bile / phlegme et à la création de la « bile noire ». C'est un raisonnement e silentio dont, il est vrai dans un cas non médical, l'utilisation serait inexacte.[60] De plus, dans l'exemple que je vais prendre, il me semble qu'on peut même montrer qu'une étiologie humorale par le phlegme est supposée.

Voici les rédactions parallèles de la première maladie décrite, au c. 1 et (sous forme partielle) au c. 12. J'ai souligné, à la suite de Jacques Jouanna, certaines correspondances entre les deux rédactions et indiqué les différences principales : la première rédaction a une étiologie humorale par le phlegme, la seconde rédaction n'a pas d'étiologie explicite, mais propose une longue thérapeutique qui est absente de la première rédaction, et dont je ne cite qu'une petite partie.

---

[59] Dans *Hippocrate. Pour une . . .*, 99, il traduisait « inflammation blanche », par opposition à « phlegme blanc » (« une inexactitude significative »). Sur la compatibilité entre les deux sens, cf. Thivel, *Cnide et . . .*, 78. Le lien entre le phlegme et le froid vient peut-être de sa mise en rapport, en qu'humeur descendant du cerveau, avec les maladies rhino-pharyngées de l'hiver, par opposition à la bile et aux maladies intestinales de l'été, ou au sang chaud des blessures : cf. Iain M. Lonie, *The Hippocratic Treatises « On Generation », « On the nature of the Child », « Diseases IV »* (Berlin/New York: Walter de Gruyter, 1981), 279.

[60] Quand Aristote, *H.A.* 1.11.493a3–4 évoque l'affection humaine appelée σταφυλή (*uvula*), et décrite dans *Maladies II* par deux fois, il utilise très vraisemblablement une version de cette description nosologique; or il choisit une description sans étiologie explicite, comparable à la version dite ancienne de *Maladies II*, peut-être en raison de la méfiance parfois sensible des philosophes à l'égard des distinctions humorales (cf. Demont, *About*... [cf. note 29], 279).

C. 1 :

⟨...⟩ Οὐρέεται πολλὸν ὅταν ὑπερθερμανθῇ κεφαλή· τήκεται γὰρ ἐν αὐτῇ τὸ φλέγμα· τηκόμενον δὲ χωρεῖ τὸ μὲν ἐς τὰς ῥῖνας, τὸ δ' ἐς τὸ στόμα, τὸ δὲ διὰ τῶν φλεβῶν αἳ ἄγουσιν ἐς τὸ αἰδοῖον· ὅταν δ' ἐς τὸ αἰδοῖον ἀφίκηται, οὐρεῖ καὶ πάσχει οἷά περ ὑπὸ στραγγουρίης. Ἀμβλυώσσουσι δ' ὅταν ἐς τὰ ἐν τοῖσιν ὀφθαλμοῖσι φλέβια ἐσέλθῃ φλέγμα· ὑδαρεστέρη τε γὰρ γίνεται ἡ ὄψις καὶ θολερωτέρη, καὶ τὸ λαμπρὸν ἐν τῷ ὀφθαλμῷ οὐχ ὁμοίως λαμπρόν ἐστιν, οὐδὲ καταφαίνεται ἐν αὐτῷ, ἣν θέλῃ ὁρᾶν ὁμοίως ὡς καὶ ὅτε λαμπρὸς καὶ καθαρὸς ἦν. Οὗτος ἐν τεσσαράκοντα ἡμέρῃσι μάλιστα ὑγιάζεται. Ἢν δὲ χρόνῳ ὕστερον πολλῷ ὑποστρέψῃ ἡ νοῦσος, τὸ δέρμα τῆς κεφαλῆς παχύνεται, καὶ τὸ ἄλλο σῶμα αἴρεται καὶ παχύνεται καὶ εὐχροεῖ. Τούτῳ τὸ φλέγμα ἐς τὰς σάρκας τρέπεται, καὶ ὑπὸ τούτου δοκεῖ παχὺς εἶναι· αἱ γὰρ σάρκες, ἅτε διάβροχοι ἐοῦσαι καὶ ἠρμέναι καὶ ἀραιότεραι, ἕλκουσιν ἐκ τῶν φλεβῶν αἷμα, καὶ διὰ τοῦτο δοκέουσιν εὔχροοι εἶναι

[Identification] ⟨ ...⟩ **[sémiologie + étiologie]** *Il y a émission d'une urine abondante* lorsque la tête est échauffée à l'excès. En effet, le phlegme se fond en elle ; et quand il se fond, il s'écoule, en partie dans les narines, en partie dans la bouche, en partie dans les vaisseaux qui mènent aux organes génitaux. Quand il parvient aux organes génitaux, le malade *urine et éprouve les symptômes de la strangurie.* Il y a amblyopie quand dans les petits vaisseaux *des yeux* pénètre du phlegme. En effet, l'organe de la vision devient plus humide et plus trouble, le brillant de l'oeil n'est plus aussi brillant et les objets, quand le malade veut regarder, n'y apparaissent pas avec autant de netteté que quand il était brillant et limpide. **[pronostic et étiologie supplémentaire]** *Ce malade guérit d'ordinaire en quarante jours.* Et si, beaucoup plus tard, *la maladie récidive*, la peau de la tête s'épaissit, le reste du corps se gonfle, prend de l'embonpoint et *une belle couleur*. Chez ce malade, le phlegme se tourne vers les chairs ; ce qui explique l'embonpoint apparent ; et les chairs, du moment qu'elles sont imbibées, gonflées et plus lâches, attirent le sang des vaisseaux ; de là vient la belle couleur apparente des malades (*Mal. II.*1, VII, 8 Li, 132–133 Jouanna).

C. 12

Νοῦσοι αἱ ἀπὸ τῶν κεφαλέων· νάρκα ἴσχει τὴν κεφαλὴν, καὶ οὐρεῖ θαμινά, καὶ τἆλλα πάσχει ἅπερ ὑπὸ στραγγουρίης· 2 οὗτος ἡμέρας ἐννέα ταῦτα πάσχει, καὶ ἢν μὲν ῥαγῇ κατὰ τὰς ῥῖνας ἢ κατὰ τὰ ὦτα ὕδωρ και πλέννα, ἀπαλλάσσεται τῆς νούσου, καὶ παύεται τῆς στραγγουρίης· οὐρεῖ δὲ ἀπόνως πολλὸν καὶ λευκὸν ἐς τὰς εἴκοσιν ἡμέρας, καὶ ἐκ τῆς κεφαλῆς ἡ ὀδύνη ἐκλείπει, καὶ ἐκ τῶν ὀφθαλμῶν ἐσορῶντι κλέπτεταί οἱ ἡ αὐγή, καὶ δοκεῖ το ἥμισυ τῶν προσώπων ὁρᾶν. Οὗτος τεσσαρακοσταῖος παντάπασι ὑγιὴς γίνεται· ἐνίοτε δὲ ὑπ' οὖν ἔστρεψεν ἡ νοῦσος ἑβδόμῳ ἔτει ἢ τεσσαρεσκαιδεκάτῳ· καὶ τὸ δέρμα οἱ παχύνεται τῆς κεφαλῆς καὶ ψαυόμενον ὑπείκει, καὶ ἀπ' ὀλίγων σιτίων ἁπαλὸς καὶ εὔχρως φαίνεται καὶ ἀκούει οὐκ ὀξέα. 3 Ὅταν οὕτως ἔχοντι ἐπιτύχῃς ἀρχομένῳ τῆϲ νούϲου πρόϲθεν ἢ ῥαγῆναι κατὰ τὰϲ ῥῖναϲ τὸ ὕδωρ καὶ κατὰ τὰ ὦτα καὶ ἔχῃ αὐτὸν ἡ περιωδυνίη, ἀποξυρήϲαντα χρὴ αὐτοῦ τὴν κεφαλὴν (...) 6 Ἢν δ' ὑποστρέψῃ ἡ νοῦϲοϲ, πυριήϲαϲ αὐτὸν ὅλον, ἐϲ αὔριον δοῦναι ἐλλέβορον πιεῖν, κἄπειτα διαλείπειν ὅϲον ἄν ϲοι δοκέῃ χρόνον, καὶ τότε τὴν κεφαλὴν καθῆραϲ, κατωτερικὸν δοὺϲ φάρμακον, καῦϲον τὴν κεφαλὴν ἐϲχάραϲ ὀκτώ, δύο μὲν παρὰ τὰ ὦτα, δύο δ' ἐν τοῖϲι κροτάφοιϲι, δύο δὲ ὄπιϲθεν τῆϲ κεφαλῆϲ ἔνθεν καὶ ἔνθεν ἐν τῇ κοτίδι, δύο ἐν τῇ ῥινὶ παρὰ τοὺϲ κανθούϲ· τὰϲ φλέβαϲ καίειν δὲ τὰϲ μὲν παρὰ τὰ ὦτα, ἔϲτ' ἂν παύϲωνται ϲφύζουϲαι· τοῖϲι δὲ ϲιδηρίοιϲι ϲφηνίϲκουϲ ποιηϲάμενοϲ, διακαίειν πλαγίαϲ τὰϲ φλέβαϲ. Ταῦτα ποιήϲαντι ὑγιείη ἐγγίνεται.

1 [**Identification**] Maladies provenant de la tête : [**sémiologie sans étiologie**] la tête est prise de torpeur ; *le malade urine fréquemment et éprouve tous les autres symptômes de la strangurie.* 2 Il éprouve ces symptômes durant neuf jours ; puis, s'il y a, par les narines ou par les oreilles, éruption d'eau et de mucus, la maladie disparaît et la strangurie cesse. Le malade évacue sans douleur une urine abondante et blanche jusqu'au terme de vingt jours ; la douleur de tête disparaît ; mais quand il regarde, la lumière se dérobe *à ses yeux* et il lui semble voir la moitié des visages. [**pronostic**] *Ce malade guérit complètement le quarantième jour. Mais il arrive parfois que la maladie récidive* la septième ou la quatorzième année ; alors la peau de la tête s'épaissit et cède au toucher ; et il suffit que le malade absorbe une petite quantité d'aliments pour que sa peau paraisse veloutée *et son teint bien coloré* ; l'ouïe n'est pas fine. 3 [extraits de la **thérapeutique**] Quand vous êtes en présence d'un tel malade, qu'il en est encore au début de sa maladie, avant l'éruption d'eau par les narines ou par les oreilles, rasez-lui la tête (...) 6 Si la maladie récidive, faites prendre au malade un bain de vapeur complet, et le lendemain donnez-lui à boire l'éllébore. Puis, après un délai laissé à votre appréciation, purgez alors la tête, donnez un évacuant par le bas, faites[61] à la tête huit escarres, deux le long des oreilles, deux aux tempes, deux derrière la tête, de chaque côté, à l'occiput, deux au nez, près du coin des yeux. Vous cautérisez les vaisseaux qui passent le long des oreilles jusqu'à ce qu'ils cessent de battre. Pour cela, donnez aux ferrements la forme de petits coins et cautérisez en traversant les vaisseaux pris obliquement. Avec ce traitement, la santé se rétablit (*Mal. II*, 12, VII, 18–22 Li, 142–145 Jouanna).

Un rapprochement, dans la seconde version, entre une partie de la thérapeutique proposée en cas de récidive, à savoir les cautérisations sur la tête, et la description hérodotéenne des cautérisations des Libyens pour lutter contre le phlegme, texte que j'ai cité au début de ma communication, semble possible. Ce type de cautérisation de la tête est une réalité bien documentée dans la médecine populaire et en particulier chez les

[61] Ou plutôt : « produisez ».

Berbères d'Afrique du nord,[62] et il n'y a aucune raison pour qu'il n'en ait pas été de même en Grèce. Le texte d'Hérodote atteste que lui-même et ses informateurs (des Grecs, et peut-être des médecins grecs, de Libye ?) interprétaient cette technique, au milieu du cinquième siècle, comme un moyen de lutter contre le phlegme. Il semble donc possible que la thérapeutique du c. 12 de *Maladies II* implique cette étiologie manifestement connue très tôt, et qu'on trouve dans le c. 1 du traité hippocratique.

Ce qui distingue le texte hippocratique par rapport aux cautérisations des Libyens selon Hérodote, c'est une technicité très supérieure (il ne s'agit pas de « laines non dégraissées », mais de « ferrements » d'une forme particulière !), technicité qui est présentée comme spécifique du médecin, à la fois pour la fabrication des ferrements et pour leur utilisation pour la production des escarres. Notons que cette technique médicale assez horrible n'est utilisée que dans les cas de « récidive » « la septième ou la quatorzième année » (!), et a un caractère exceptionnel, à la différence de l'usage attribué généralement aux Libyens chez Hérodote. Dans le cas de *Maladies II*, on est donc en présence d'une technique qui a des aspects très anciens, largement attestés dans les médecines traditionnelles, mais qui est intégrée dans un corpus médical élaboré, avec des raffinements techniques, comme une solution de dernier recours, et qui reçoit dès le milieu du cinquième siècle une explication humorale en rapport avec les différentes systématisations progressives des humeurs au sein de la médecine hippocratique.

Dans cet exposé ont été soulignées les difficultés de l'interprétation de la *Collection hippocratique* et de l'évaluation de l'ancienneté relative de ses descriptions nosologiques. Chemin faisant, place a été faite à différentes façons (le sujet pourrait être développé) qu'avaient les médecins hippocratiques de construire, dès la période classique, l'histoire de leur art, en élargissant ou en restreignant le domaine de la médecine, en opposant la médecine diététique à la médecine traditionnelle, ou encore en attestant la réalité d'une construction collective et progressive, dans la com-

---

[62] Cf. Althoff, *Herodot und* ..., 9–10 et Thomas, *Herodotus in* ..., 36. Je remercie Luc Renaut de ses observations sur les parallèles ethnographiques. Il a déjà proposé le rapprochement entre le texte d'Hérodote et celui de *Maladies II* dans son article sur « Les tatouages d'Ötzi et la petite chirurgie traditionnelle », *L'anthropologie* 108 (2004): 69–105 (voir notamment p. 93, avec aussi un utile renvoi à Marie-Hélène Marganne, *L'ophtalmologie dans l'Egypte grécoromaine d'après les papyrus littéraires grecs*, (Leiden: Brill, 1994), 147–172, pour les cautérisations en cas de fluxions oculaires).

pétition multiforme entre médecins et groupes de médecins qui caractérise sans aucun doute possible l'état de cette profession dans la Grèce, et dans l'Orient, à l'époque classique. Que cette compétition les ait amenés à rivaliser avec leurs collègues et prédécesseurs babyloniens est fort vraisemblable, mais c'est là une autre histoire, qui conduira certainement les hellénistes à modifier leurs perspectives.

SOURCE INDEX

Near Eastern Sources

Classical Sources

AKKADIAN AND SUMERIAN WORDS TREATED

GENERAL INDEX